OPI

N

OPHTHALMIC NURSING

A Samuel Gnanadoss
BA, BD, MS, DO, FIAMS, PGDHM
Senior Consultant
Arasan Eye Hospital
26, Annamalai Layout
Erode, Tamil Nadu
India

JAYPEE BROTHERS MEDICAL PUBLISHERS (P) LTD

Chennai • St Louis (USA) • Panama City (Panama) • London (UK) • New Delhi
Ahmedabad • Bengaluru • Hyderabad • Kochi • Kolkata • Lucknow • Mumbai • Nagpur

Published by

Jitendar P Vij

Jaypee Brothers Medical Publishers (P) Ltd

Corporate Office

4838/24 Ansari Road, Daryaganj, **New Delhi** - 110002, India, Phone: +91-11-43574357
Fax: +91-11-43574314

Registered Office

B-3 EMCA House, 23/23B Ansari Road, Daryaganj, **New Delhi** - 110 002, India
Phones: +91-11-23272143, +91-11-23272703, +91-11-23282021
+91-11-23245672, Rel: +91-11-32558559, Fax: +91-11-23276490, +91-11-23245683
e-mail: jaypee@jaypeebrothers.com, Website: www.jaypeebrothers.com

Offices in India

- **Ahmedabad,** Phone: Rel: +91-79-32988717, e-mail: ahmedabad@jaypeebrothers.com
- **Bengaluru,** Phone: Rel: +91-80-32714073, e-mail: bangalore@jaypeebrothers.com
- **Chennai,** Phone: Rel: +91-44-32972089, e-mail: chennai@jaypeebrothers.com
- **Hyderabad,** Phone: Rel:+91-40-32940929, e-mail: hyderabad@jaypeebrothers.com
- **Kochi,** Phone: +91-484-2395740, e-mail: kochi@jaypeebrothers.com
- **Kolkata,** Phone: +91-33-22276415, e-mail: kolkata@jaypeebrothers.com
- **Lucknow,** Phone: +91-522-3040554, e-mail: lucknow@jaypeebrothers.com
- **Mumbai,** Phone: Rel: +91-22-32926896, e-mail: mumbai@jaypeebrothers.com
- **Nagpur,** Phone: Rel: +91-712-3245220, e-mail: nagpur@jaypeebrothers.com

Overseas Offices

- **North America Office, USA,** Ph: 001-636-6279734
  e-mail: jaypee@jaypeebrothers.com, anjulav@jaypeebrothers.com
- **Central America Office, Panama City, Panama,** Ph: 001-507-317-0160
  e-mail: cservice@jphmedical.com
  Website: www.jphmedical.com
- **Europe Office, UK,** Ph: +44 (0) 2031708910, e-mail: info@jpmedpub.com

Ophthalmic Nursing

© 2010, Jaypee Brothers Medical Publishers (P) Ltd.

First Edition: **2010**

ISBN 978-93-80704-11-1

Typeset at JPBMP typesetting unit
Printed at Sanat Printers, Kundli.

I dedicate this book to my two lovely children,
Martha Satya and Marcus Abraham,
who encouraged me to plunge into writing this book

PREFACE

The very fact that eye is receiving 90% of sensory impulses from the outside world underscores its importance. This also means that a nurse dealing with eye patients occupies a strategic place. At the same time, while dealing with such a delicate organ, a small mistake committed by her—whether it be in the outpatient section, ward or operation theatre—may result in devastating effect on the eye and vision.

The ophthalmic nurse must know about various eye conditions, must have a thorough knowledge of the various equipment and must be an exceptionally good nurse knowing all the aspects of ophthalmic nursing.

Having worked in India and abroad as ophthalmologist for the last four decades and having taken classes for nurses, I have seen what a good nurse means to the surgeon and what catastrophe an inefficient nurse can cause. It should be the aim of all nurses to achieve that diadem of efficiency.

This work endeavours to achieve these aims. At the same time, a nurse should constantly update herself with the various advances made in ophthalmic field. This book can form that foundation for such advancement.

While writing this book I have kept in mind the Indian nurses. But at the same time I have not forgotten to include those advances made abroad which are sure to percolate into India soon.

If nurses—students and working—find this book useful to them, then my efforts are rewarded and my aim in writing this book is achieved.

I have used the 'she' for nurses and 'he' for patients. This system I have followed for convenience. This can never mean that there are no male nurses and that there are no female patients!

A Samuel Gnanadoss

ACKNOWLEDGEMENTS

I am grateful to Dr Kalavathy, Deputy Director of Dr Joseph Eye Hospital, Trichy, Dr N Rajendran, Professor of Ophthalmology, Tutucorin Medical College and Dr Dhinukumar Arthur, Associate Professor of Ophthalmology for the excellent photographs they provided for this book.

I am deeply indebted to Dr Ratnaraj Arthur, Ophthalmic Surgeon of Pondicherry, for his help.

I must thank my computerists, N Sundaranathan and V Arunkumar, and technician Sundararaman for their assistance.

Most of the line diagrams have been drawn by me. They may lack the artistic touch. But it is my desire that they should be scientifically accurate. Appasamy Associates (instrument manufacturers of Chennai) have kindly permitted me to use many of their pictures for which I am duty bound to thank them.

My gratitude to my wife Leela is great for putting up with all the inconveniences I caused to her while preparing this manuscript and leaving me all alone with my academic pursuit.

Last but not the least, I am duty bound to thank Jaypee Brothers Medical Publishers (P) Ltd., especially Mr Tarun Duneja and Mr Jayanandan, for their useful suggestions and encouragement they gave me when I wrote this book.

CONTENTS

CHAPTER

1

History of
Nursing

INTRODUCTION

Nursing encompasses autonomous and collaborative care of individuals of all ages, families, groups and communities, sick or well and in all settings. Nursing includes the promotion of health, prevention of illness, and the care of ill, disabled and dying people. Advocacy, promotion of a safe environment, research, participation in shaping health policy and in patient and health systems management, and education are also key nursing roles.

"The use of clinical judgement in the provision of care to enable people to improve, maintain, or recover health, to cope with health problems, and to achieve the best possible quality of life, whatever their disease or disability, until death".

Definition

Nursing is the promotion, and optimization of health and abilities; prevention of illness or injury; alleviation suffering through the diagnosis and treatment of human responses; and advocacy in health care for individuals, families, communities, and populations.

BEFORE THE COMMON ERA

Nursing has existed in various forms in every culture, although the definition of the term and the practice of nursing have changed greatly over time. The oldest sense of the word in the English language is found from the 14th century and referred to a woman employed to suckle and generally care a younger child. The former being known as a wet nurse and the latter being known as a dry nurse.

Prehistoric people suffered similar conditions to what are suffered today. The early humans may have taken part in the care of the sick. At the 'home' it was often the female relatives who would do the day-to-day care tasks and hence she ought to have been the nurse in ancient times.

Early manuscripts on nursing focus on the role of children's nursemaids and wet nurses, roles carried out exclusively by women. The sick were cared for at home. There is some evidence that the professions of nursing and midwifery have existed for many years in some form or other.

One of the earliest references to women as "Nurses" is to be found in the Bible (about 500 BC) and this information might have been from older sources, may be as early as 800 BC.

Further evidence suggests that midwives had a similar role to those of today, in assisting with birth.

These midwives/nurses also knew the arts of bandaging, dressing, use of oil, wine and balsam and had rules of diet and used purgatives. Not only did they care for the ill, but they performed operations, administered sleeping draughts, made artificial limbs and carried out isolation to prevent infections from spreading.

Eastern civilizations were ahead of the west in understanding and caring for health. According to Susruta, the code of surgical nursing forbids the services of a female nurse; even the sight of a female is undesirable. Emperor Asoka of northern India (around 225 BC) built 18 hospitals (and medical schools) in which older women and men nursed patients.

In Homer's Iiiad, a story written around 1,300 BC, is the first recorded women nurse: Hekamede. She was to wash away the clotted blood on the battlefield. The Greeks believed that Asklepios' two sons and six daughters were famed in the arts of healing. Still it is doubtful that women would have played an important role in caring for the sick. There were priestesses at the altars, women orderlies who directed the bath attendants and porters, and midwives; however, women were of no great account among the Greeks at this time. In the battle fields nursing was undertaken of the wounded by trained nurses who could anticipate the doctor's desire for necessary information – perhaps an early indication that nursing was led by the medical profession – and these were probably women. Hippocrates omitted any discussion of nurse training. Women midwives (omphalotomai-navel cutters) at this time were also common, but not trained and did not work with doctors.

Slave girls assisted the Roman physicians who were also slaves. As the empire grew hospitals were built, some of which could admit up to 200 patients (one hospital for every three legions). Most of the nurses would have been men called conttubernalis (tent companion – from the time when field hospitals were in tents). Roman soldiers were also taught first aid to enable them to nurse their comrades on the battle field.

In Coluella, a civilian hospital (valetudinarium), the Bailiff's wife was instructed to keep the valetudinarium clean, to air the wards so that the sick would find their rooms healthy, and watch over the ill. Fabiola a wealthy Roman woman devoted her life for the sick (Fig. 1.1). By the time of her death in 399, Fabiola had made nursing the sick and poor fashionable in Roman society.

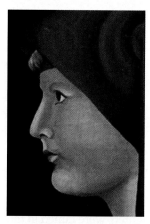

Figure 1.1: Fabiola

At this time, in cities, towns and villages, care was not organized. There were many quacks and charlatans. Alice Shevyngon, a maidservant left her master and took to curing people with sore eye. It appears the 'ophthalmic nursing' was more profitable for Alice. Nursing became fashionable; but the Church insisted that the way to cure was through prayer and fasting, asking for the help of saints and belief in miracles. The new aristocratic nurses relied on divine help as did the nuns, built hospitals and worked in them as nurses. Queen Matilda, or Maud, wife of Henry I (1110) carried on the nursing tradition, founding hospital for lepers in London.

During the reformation period many 'heretics' were burnt as witches, including uncloistered monks and nuns, who cared for the sick. This period also saw Knight Tempellar, who were mostly warriors, look after the sick and suffering (Fig. 1.2).

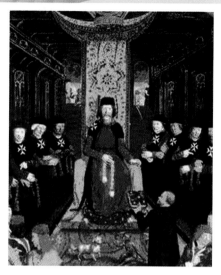

Figure 1.2: Knights Tempellar

Without the nuns (expelled from their convents and aristocratic interest dwindling) the character of nursing changed. Nuns were replaced by local women and the Mother Superior by 'Matron' who was responsible for the 'sister' and to see they did their work properly. Most of these duties were domestic.

Camillus de Lellis, a priest born at Bucchianico, Abruzzi, Italy, in 1550 became the patron Saint of Nurses.

Nurses Pay

By 1700 two types of people worked in the hospitals—paid and unpaid. Pay was low, with the Matron getting cash and the nurses being paid in a variety of other ways, such as bread and beer. It is not surprising that some nurses took money from patients without considering it as being wrong.

During 1837-1901 St. Thomas Hospital paid its sisters 37 pounds per year and nurses 25. At St. George's hospital sisters were paid 21 pounds and nurses 16. Everyone got six pounds of bread a week, two pints of table beer daily and a shilling a day for board and wages. At Guy's hospital, to help prevent the nurses taking the patients' money, sisters were paid 50 pounds per year and nurses 30. Nurses pay was equivalent to a cotton operative and a sisters no better than an untrained teacher.

NURSING IN THE ARMED FORCES

The army nursing service began in a limited way after Crimea war (1854 – 1856) when the first female trained nurses were attached to the Army Medical school Hospitals, first at Netley then at Woolwich. The service was reorganized after the Boer War (1899 – 1902) under the patronage of Queen Alexandra (wife of Edward VII) and became the Queen Alexandra Imperial Military Nursing Service. After the First World War, the royal Air Force developed its own medical service to which was attached the princess Mary Royal Air Force Nursing Service.

NURSING IN INDIA

The first nursing school in the world was started in India in about 250 BC. Only men were considered "pure" enough to become nurses. The Charaka states these men should be, "of good behaviour, distinguished for purity, possessed of cleverness and skill imbued with kindness, skilled in every service a patient may require, competent to cook food, skilled in bathing and washing the patient, rubbing and massaging the limbs".

The Indian mutiny in India of 1857 prompted Nightingale that care of the soldiers is a must. It was for this purpose the Royal Commission was appointed in 1859. In 1868, a sanitary department was established. In March 1888, ten qualified British nurses arrived in India to look after the British Army in India. In 1905, during the British rule in India, missionary nurses arrived as members of Missionary Medical Association. This was the very start of formalized nursing service in India. Gradually, the increasing need of adequately trained nurses led to creation of South India Examining Board in 1911 and the North India Examining Board in 1912. It was the mission hospital nursing leaders who laid the foundation of systematic Nursing education in India. State-wise councils started developing from 1935 onwards and by 2001, 19 State-wise registration councils came into existence. Indian Nursing Council (INC) Act was passed by the Parliament in 1947. The Nursing Council upgraded the educational requirements which permitted only matriculated candidates to seek admission to the schools.

The Central Government granted an approval to the Bhore Committee's (1946) recommendations by starting two colleges of Nursing in Delhi (1946) and Vellore (1947). This provided university degree level courses. With the efforts of Professor S. Radhakrishnan (the then Chairman of University Education Commission), Nursing education in the country was integrated into the system of higher education.

TOWARDS REGISTRATION

It was in the area of mental health that the first nationally recognized qualifications came in existence. Other opposition came from hospital administrators and doctors who thought that 'newfangled registered nurses' would 'eat into' some of their livelihood.

In 1902, because of the concern about the deaths of women in childbirth, it was decided that midwives should be registered with a central board. The supporters of nurse registration saw this as an opportunity to persuade the government to set up a committee to investigate the registration of nurses. The committee agreed in principle but recommended two registers, one for those with a complete training and one for the less highly trained–a proposal implemented nearly 40 years later.

The early days were stormy with disagreements between the government and profession about the standards required for registration and which hospitals should be accepted as training hospitals.

New Zealand was the first country to regulate nurses nationally, with adoption of the Nurses Registration Act on the 12th of September, 1901. Ellen Dougherty was the first Registered Nurse. North Carolina was the first state in the United States to pass a nursing licensure law in 1903.

FLORENCE NIGHTINGALE (FIG. 1.3)

She was the second daughter of William Edward Nightingale and Frances Smith. She was educated largely by her father. Throughout her life she read widely in many languages. On Feb 7, 1837 she believed that she had heard the voice of God informing her that she had a mission, but it was not until nine years later that she realized what the mission was.

In 1846, a friend sent Nightingale the Year Book of the Institution of Protestant Deaconesses at Kaiserswerth, Germany, which trained country girls of good character to nurse the sick. Four years later she entered the institution and went through the full course of training as a nurse. In 1853 she was appointed superintendent of the Institution for the care of Sick Gentlewomen, in London.

The Crimean war broke out in March 1854, and the British were dismayed by the disgraceful conditions suffered by sick and wounded British soldiers. Nightingale volunteered at once and left in three days for Constantinople, taking three nurses with her. The

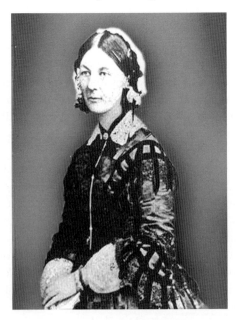

Figure 1.3: Florence Nightingale

party left England on Oct. 21, 1854, and entered the barrack Hospital at Scutari on November 5. She changed the whole face of nursing and the battle field hospital.

After the war Nightingale returned to England. But she refused official transport home and every kind of public reception. The Indian mutiny turned Nightingale's interest to the health of the army in India, and for that purpose another royal commission was appointed in 1859. This resulted in 1868 in the establishment of a sanitary Department in the India office.

From 1857 Nightingale had lived, mainly in London, as an invalid. It has never been shown that Florence Nightingale had any organic illness; her invalidism may have been partly neurotic and partly intentional. Her sight gradually failed and in 1901 she became completely blind. In 1907 the king conferred on her the Order of Merit – the first woman ever to receive it. Florence Nightingale died in 1910.

Other important nurses in the development of the profession include: Mary Seacole, who also worked as a nurse in the Crimea; Agnes Elizabeth Jones and Linda Richards, who established quality nursing schools in the USA and Japan, and Linda Richards who was officially America's First Trained Nurse.

2

Ophthalmic Nurse and the Patient

A nurse has to deal with varied situations and varieties of patients in ophthalmology unlike other branches of nursing.

PATIENTS

They present a kaleidoscopic picture. But mostly they are a worried lot. Eye being the organ receiving 90% of stimuli from external world, and as most of its diseases being very obvious, it is natural that the patient is worried. He may be deeply apprehensive and may need reassurance repeatedly. The attending surgeon will be able to explain the eye condition and assure the patient that all is well. But it is the nurse who has to provide that courage to the patient, sometimes repeatedly.

While dealing with patients going for surgery, she must be well versed with the operative procedure and the instructions that should be given. She must emphasise to the patient the importance of them. Many patients do not take these instructions seriously endangering the precious eyes.

AGE

The ophthalmic patient can be of any age and belong to extremes of age. The patience of a nurse is required while dealing with a crying, uncooperative new born or a child, and with a very aged whose mental faculty might have gone down so much that he may even be unaware of what is happening around him. The aged may forget the instructions that are given to him so that he may have to be repeatedly told patiently.

RELATIVES

The relatives can sometimes be as demanding as the patient himself. Their apprehension is well justified especially if the patient is a child. They may be worried to the extreme and they may need as much assurance as the patient.

Relatives of an aged patient can be a heterogeneous set. They can range from "we don't care" type to extremely inquisitive and worried set. In many homes, the aged may have crossed the earning capacity and they may be looked upon by the relatives as a burden. When such a patient is brought, the nurse may find unattached relatives to deal with. On the other hand, in some homes the aged may be looked upon as some semi-God by the family members. The attendants of such patient may sometimes tax upon the patience of the nurse.

What ever may be the situation, the nurse has to be patient with the relatives as much as she is with the patient. Many a time the instructions may have to be given to the relative.

PROCEDURES

It is almost wholly left to the nurse to explain to the patient any procedure that might be carried out. It may be a very minor one as removal of conjunctival foreign body or a major one such as retinal detachment surgery. It may be a non operative one such as laser application or tonometry. The nurse herself must have knowledge of the instruments, the procedure itself and the various "discomfort" and side effects it can cause. She must make the patient completely relaxed and infuse confidence in him.

She must elicit history of other diseases – especially in older people. This is important since a diabetic or severe hypertensive should not be made to wait in the outpatient for long.

EYE CONDITION

Some patient may be philosophical in their attitude towards his disease; while others might be very agitated. The nurse must calm down the latter and inculcate into the mind of the former to take their eye condition seriously.

Day surgical cases have to be specially looked after since they may not have much time to adjust and the nurse also may not have much time with them. They may need information about their disease and about the operation which are to be done. She must use simple language. Use of charts will be more helpful. Instruction leaflet is useful and negates repetition of instructions to patient as well as to his relatives.

The *visual loss* or defect varies. Persons with good acuity of vision but having serious eye problem (such as open angle glaucoma, papilledema and retinitis pigmentosa) must be tactfully informed about the gravity of situation without alarming them. Support those with permanent blindness/defective vision/night blindness emotionally. They need this. Consider each case as a person and not as being made up of eye only.

Once the patient with irreversible blindness has finished his consultation, assure him that he still can lead a normal life with the help of *rehabilitation*. Provide him with address of the organisation where it is available. For those with diseases of relentless progress (such as retinitis pigmentosa) show them the silver lining in the dark cloud.

Trauma cases need special care. They are already upset about the accident and about the state of eye condition. Nurse must reassure them; but should not give too much of hope. Nurse should not be callous to a patient who attends the casualty with only lid swelling. As far as the patient is concerned, it is a disease.

The nurse must be very gentle and understanding. The eye is a delicate organ. A closed eye may have a grave problem inside (such as rupture globe) which might worsen and result in loss of eye if forcibly opened.

As talking to patient is the most important aspect, the nurse must know the local *language*. This is very important in India which has 14 major languages.

The nurse must have up-to-date *knowledge of* basic ophthalmology. She must be well versed with all the latest ophthalmic instruments and gadgets. She must be able to maintain these equipments and must know the basic working of them. She must be able to record vision and carry out minor checking.

She must correctly and in detail tell the *instructions* to the patient and, if patient belongs to extremes of age, to the relatives. But when the patient leaves the ward / O.P his relatives must have completely understood the instructions. There are instances (as reported by the great physician Albert Schweitzer) of patients eating the eye ointment rather than applying it. She must constantly assess herself, study the mistakes she has made and improve herself.

A word of caution about *false beliefs*. Superstition and false beliefs are very much ingrained in people's minds throughout the world. In India it is more. A nurse must have the tact and the persuasion capacity while dealing with this aspect. It is very difficult to convince people that they are having false ideas. Worse is, some tend to consider that the surgeon/nurse is no good and does not know the subject well. But health education on this aspect is a must to remove such dangerous practices and beliefs from the people. Application of milk, leaf juice and oil to the eye is a common practice. For instance, small pox virus does not invade the cornea very much. But in previous generation blindness due to corneal scar in small pox cases was common. This is mostly due to application of irritants to the eyes. This stems from the popular false belief that a patient should not be unconscious and should be awakened by applying irritants to the eye.

An ophthalmic nurse may be *posted in* a) outpatient, b) ward or in c) operation theatre. Usually to be a theatre nurse, it needs special training. Basically devotion is needed.

Out Patient

The nurse must be the first person to arrive at the outpatient section in the morning. She has to see to the cleanliness of the whole outpatient section. The equipments have to be kept ready for the day's work. The registers and other documents have to be in place. She must see that other paramedical personnel are at their duty spot by the time the first patient arrives. Punctuality and discipline are needed, as out patient is where patients flock and their relatives observe the working of the hospital staff.

Minor procedures are carried out and instruments for the same must be sterilized and kept ready. The nurse must have a good knowledge of these procedures and the underlying reason for performing them.

She must devote some time with the patients who are for *admission*. She must be able to elicit proper history from the patient, especially about any systemic disease he has. She must see that the proper investigations are carried out. She need not get all tests done. They should be based on indications and risk factors. Tests needed for anaesthetist must be done even if the case is for operation under local anaesthesia. Blood grouping and cross matching are required for cases posted for major surgeries such as exenteration. Focus of infection must be checked and necessary material for microbiological tests sent.

Jewellery should be removed and *tilak* (the dot on the forehead) must be removed or (in married women) put on the neck. Nurse should confirm that the patient has understood all the preoperative instructions. If needed she must ask the patients to repeat them. If possible she must use audiovisual method. She must encourage the patient. She must send ALL cases for anaesthesia assessment. Dietary advise must be given. She must get his informed consent signed.

In the out patient location she may not be able to devote much attention to each patient. She must scan the outpatient crowd and pay special attention to those who are perplexed. She must be able to properly guide the patients to various sections, explain what these sections are for and when they come out clear any doubts they might have. She must pay special attention to those who are deeply perturbed about the poor prognosis that has been pronounced by the doctor for their eye condition. She cannot afford to be ignorant of the eye diseases. She must have basic knowledge of all eye diseases and a good knowledge of common eye conditions and their treatment.

Day-case surgery is now followed much and in western countries more than half the cases are done as day-case surgeries. The commonest major operation done this way is cataract surgery. Others include corneal transplant, eye lid and lacrymal apparatus surgery, squint and refractive surgeries. The selection of cases depends on following *criteria* and a nurse must assist the doctor in selecting day-case surgery: a) Surgical criteria – Routine surgery, surgery of about 60 minutes and less and cases in whom major complications are not expected. b) Medical criteria – Risk I and II of anaesthesia, medically fit cases and patient who is not pregnant. c) Availability of conveyance, communication and escort.

Patient must be given the date of surgery. Correct and proper preoperative instructions must be told. Cleanliness must be emphasized. IOL calculation and other investigations (local and systemic) must be completed. The usual problems he might encounter (about which he need not worry) after surgery and about certain symptoms for which he must seek immediate remedy from the doctor must be told.

The *details of the out patient cases* must be recorded. These are necessary later for statistical purpose, for research, for morbidity survey and, rarely, for legal purposes. All records must be preserved.

At the *end of the day* she must be the last to leave the out patient section. All documents should be stacked in proper places. She must check that all the instruments are cleaned, sent for sterilisation (if needed), and next day's linen is packed and dispatched for sterilisation.

Casuality work is almost same as the OPD work except for its urgency, the need for immediate treatment/surgery and the necessity for quite a lot of assurance to patient and to the relatives. *Triage* procedure is employed by the nurse in screening the cases. In this procedure the patients are divided by nurse into a) emergency cases (Sudden severe loss of vision, trauma with open eye globe, chemical burns and corneal foreign body), b) Urgent cases (gradual loss of vision, flashes of light, glaring, diplopia, blunt trauma to eye) and c) routine cases (eye discharge, irritation of eye, problem with near vision).

In casualty *investigations* ordered must be immediately carried out for emergency cases.

The nurse in casualty must have knowledge of *first aid* for eye injuries. An alkali burn case cannot wait for the ophthalmologist on duty and treatment of open globe needs immediate attention (such as antibiotic and patching).

Emergency Care

No eye emergency is so grave and no eye emergency is so simple. A simple case may present with urgent symptoms; while a patient with serious emergency may be calm. But nurse should never neglect any case.

If it is a case of chemical splash (acid or alkali) to the eye, irrigate eye INSTANTANEOUSLY with any fluid – even tap water. Time should not be wasted in searching for kidney tray, saline, irrigation pump, etc.

For other cases, local patching with antibiotic ointment should be done till the ophthalmologist arrives. The nurse should be guarded against patient with acute catarrhal conjunctivitis – they will swear that some foreign body has fallen into the eye. Eye patch should be avoided in such cases and irrigation of eye should be done with saline. It is better for the eye surgeon to examine such cases to exclude foreign body.

Ward

Compared to outpatient duty, the ward work may not be so crowded. But the work is equally responsible. With the advent of day surgery, the work load and number of in-patients have come down.

Nurse must always be at duty spot in the ward and should maintain the duty timing. She is wholly in charge of the ward. Safety and maintenance of equipments, linen and documents are her responsibility.

The *ward* must be clean and properly maintained. Room spray can be used. The ward should be quiet. Special attention must be paid to illumination especially during the night hours. The toilet must be clean and should be able to cater to the needs of the partially sighted.

The *doctor's orders* (which should be duly signed by him) ought to be carried out promptly and on time. Oral instructions given by doctors about medications should be followed. If the doctor's instructions are not legible, it is better for the nurse to clarify them with him rather than assume something and end up doing the wrong thing. If systemic medication is advised, the nurse should be sure whether it is oral, intravenous or intramuscular. The dose and frequency must be clearly indicated. Nurse chart must contain the time (entered accurately) of administration of drugs, the dose and route given and other procedures carried out. Proper handing over and taking over between nurses changing duties are important.

Instructions for cases going in *for operation* should be strictly followed. The identification tags carefully checked and tied. The patient, his records and any drug that might be needed during surgery (including IOL) must be sent with him to operation theatre (OT) in time. The patient should be reassured. His doubts must be cleared. His signature in informed consent form must be obtained.

When the patient comes back from the operation theatre, she has to check his case record, diligently follow the post operative instructions contained therein. Again assure him that all is well. His pulse, BP, temperature and respiration rate must be recorded.

If the nurse is posted in *day-case surgery unit,* she must admit him in the unit, check the BP, pulse, temperature and confirm that he has come on empty stomach. Sedation is avoided as the patient has to go home after surgery. If it is absolutely required, oral midazolam is used. She should check all the biochemical results.

At the time of *discharge* from the hospital, the nurse must properly advise the patient (operated and others) about what he should do and should not do, what medicines he should take and how they should be taken. He also must be told when and where he should come for review. He should have the emergency number of the hospital. The discharge card must contain all important details. The idea of rest for one month after cataract operation is gone. It is now early return to normal life. At the same time caution must be exercised. There are certain cataracts—IOL surgeons who say that one can do cooking the same day. This is overstepping the limits of caution and some patients may go beyond this limit also. With modern cataract surgery using rollable IOL, a person can attend to his work the very next day as long as there is no heavy exertion or dusty atmosphere.

Strict instruction must be given about local eye drops and the way it should be applied. Local drops must be continued for one month for cases who have undergone intraocular surgery.

The completeness of patient's in-patient record must be assessed and sent to medical records section.

Comatose patients need special and careful attention. Severe cases may not be in eye ward. But when a nurse encounters such a case in ICU she must give diligent care to the patient's eyes.

1. The most important attention is to prevent setting in of exposure keratitis (a kind of corneal ulcer). Antibiotic ointment or artificial tear should be applied frequently in the eye. Except antibiotic ointment, nothing else should be applied in the eyes. Cortisone eye ointment should not be used.
2. Mydriatic should not be used as pupillary reaction is an important sign for the general physician/surgeon.
3. Cleaning of the eye is done with saline and eye lids should be wiped from inside (from nasal to temporal side) to out side canthi.
4. The lids must be kept closed. This is achieved by patching the eye or by a plaster attached to upper lid and to the check (after pulling down the upper lid). In both the instances care should be taken that the cornea is not damaged by the patch or by the plaster. Covering the eye is more important if the corneal reflex is absent.
5. Eyes should be checked up frequently for redness of conjunctiva, corneal ulceration or presence of pus.

SAFETY OF NURSES

All the health care personnel (which include the nurses) are liable to some injury of some form or other. They have to guard themselves against these.

I. *Infection:* The danger of infection is ever present for the nurses. It can occur in the out patient section, in the wards and in the operation theater (OT). Nurse must always clean her hands before and after handling a patient, especially if it is an infectious disease case. She must always wear gloves while dealing with such cases. This also prevents cross infection to the patient.

In case there has occurred contact with infected case/material, the nurse must immediately take the necessary steps such as antibiotics.

II. *Injuries:* These are also present everywhere. She may be injured by the equipments she might be using. Prevention and carefulness are more important. If such an accident occurs, she must take appropriate treatment. She must be careful while dealing with electrical appliances. If there is any doubt she must call in the qualified electrician and not try anything herself.

The nurse can be injured by the sterilisers she handles. Ethylene dioxide is a cancer causing agent. It should not come in contact with skin. It should not be inhaled. Formaldehyde is toxic to respiratory tract. It is an allergy producing and cancer causing agent. It can affect liver. Glutaraldehyde fumes may irritate the eye and nose. Ultra violet irradiation can cause skin burns and conjunctivitis.

Lasers are useful but dangerous equipments. Careless meddling with laser equipment should be avoided and it is better the staff learns about laser instrument first and even then it is better if she uses it under supervision only.

III. *Legal:* With modern day awareness by the patients and their relatives, a nurse and her team must guard against legal entangling. She must always get the informed consent for any case which goes for surgery of any kind. If the patient is dangerously ill, she must get the "dangerously ill (DIL)" form signed by the relatives. Proper and detailed documents are the best protection of medical team.

Finally a word about the *nurse herself*—she must be professional and kind. She must avoid excess make up or glamorous dressing. The uniform must be clean and personal hygiene must be attended to since ophthalmic work involves close quarter dealing. Bad breath and body odor must not be present. An ophthalmic nurse should not have long finger nail. She must properly tie her hair.

CERTAIN TERMS

Following are certain terms used for those who deal with eye:

Ophthalmologist: Also called ophthalmic surgeon or oculist; he is the doctor who treats all diseases of eye.

Optician: He is not a doctor. He prepares, fixes and dispenses lenses (for spectacles).

Optometrist: He examines and prescribes glasses. He does not use medicines for treating eye diseases. He does not prepare (spectacle) glasses.

Ophthalmic assistant: He is a person who is trained to diagnose and treat simple eye diseases. He assists doctors in camps and sometimes in simple operations.

Orthoptist: He deals with visual disorders especially of infants and children with muscle disorders and imbalance.

Ocularist: He measures and fits patients with prosthesis such as shell or artificial eyes.

3

Procedures

It is very difficult to differentiate out patient ("minor") and in-patient ("major") procedures in ophthalmology. It is a question of whether it is based on the time taken for the surgery or its impact on the vision. Perhaps, procedures done in out patient department can be considered as minor procedures. Here again the dispute cannot be so easily solved. For example, centres differ about where to operate on pterygium and lacrymal sac. One can take for granted that any incisional surgery as "major" procedure and others (including laser application) as "minor" procedure.

DRUG APPLICATION

Equipment needed
1. Clean tray with drugs
2. Sterile gloves
3. Sterile cotton ball (moist)
4. Kidney tray
5. For sub conjunctival injection – 2 cc syringe, 24 G needle and 2% lignocaine drops
6. Materials needed for patching (bandaging) the eye.
   - Before applying a drug the nurse must carefully check whether it is ophthalmic preparation, the name – the pharmacological rather than the propriety name, its strength and the expiry date of the drug. The name on the container must be compared with the doctor's order at least twice. Medicine from a bottle or tube which has no label on it should never be used.
   - The nurse must be sure that she is dealing with the correct patient. The eye in which the drug has to be instilled must be properly verified. Many centers use the terms OD, OS and OU for right, left and both eyes respectively.
   - The foremost importance is absolute cleanliness. The rack (or container) in which the medicines are kept must be clean. She must wash her hands before and after application. Sterile gloves must be worn.
   - The patient may be seated or lying down. She must tell the patient what she is going to do. She should clean the lids of all discharge and dirt with sterile cotton balls. If possible she

must carefully clean the pus from conjunctiva, if it is present. Cornea should not be scratched. The patient is given a cotton ball to wipe any drop that might flow over the check.

- Cornea is the most sensitive part in the human body and hence any ointment or drop should not be applied over it. Dropper bottle or ointment nozzle should be kept 2 cm above the eye. It must be applied in the conjunctival sac of lower fornix by pulling down the lower lid with the thumb placed on check bone (Fig. 3.1). The patient must be asked to look up (at the ceiling). When the patient closes the eye or blinks, the drug gets diffused over the cornea. Approach the eye from the side. This should be followed even for corneal condition.

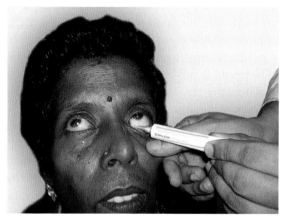

Figure 3.1: Ointment application. About 2 cm of ointment is applied from inner to outer side of the eye. The tip of nozzle should not touch the lid or the eyelash

- Ointment dispensed in applicaps form is the ideal one as it prevents cross infection. If drops are used then the first drop and, if it is ointment, the first blob are discarded. Medication of another person should not be used. If, in out-patient, an ointment tube has to be used for many patients, then the ointment is squeezed on a sterile blunt glass rod, and with the help of the latter the ointment is applied in the patient's eye.
- If it is desired that the drug should act longer or if the drug is not to be absorbed into the body through nose, the lacrymal sac area is pressed for 30 seconds after drug application.

After application the eye lids should not be squeezed. If necessary eye can be patched.

- If the drug is in suspension form and not in solution, then the container should be shaken well before the medicine is applied to the eye.
- Patients should be tutored about side effects of the drug, especially if they are going to use it at home. They must be aware of the allergic reactions or toxic effects. After application the patient must be observed for 5 minutes. If local anaesthetic drops have been instilled, then the patient must be told that he may not feel any foreign body falling in the eye for the next 30 minutes.
- When patients are advised to use drops at home they must be given proper instructions especially about cleanliness. Some patients are able to apply drops themselves while others may need someone to do it. In the latter case, the relative must be properly advised. Travatan dosing aid monitors the time when the drops are applied. (This device is now restricted to antiglaucoma medication).
- Subconjunctival injection is another method of administering drugs to the eye. One should be careful while giving this injection. There are many instances of needle penetrating the globe and the injection given inside the eye. The eye can be lost also. Local anaesthetic drop is instilled. A small fold of conjunctiva is picked up near lower fornix with a non toothed forceps and the injection given under this fold.
- All relevant data, especially the side reactions observed, must be documented and patient warned.

IRRIGATION OF EYE

Equipment needed –
1. Sterile irrigation fluid in the bulb syringe
2. Anaesthetic drops
3. Sterile gloves
4. Sterile cotton balls
5. Kidney tray

6. Drape.
7. Eye patch, if needed

The washing of the eye (this is the term commonly used; but it is not the eye, but mainly the conjunctiva and cornea that are washed) is done with normal saline. If distilled water is used, patient may have irritation as the distilled water surface tension will differ from that of tear that is normally present over the conjunctiva and cornea.

- Nurse must explain to the patient what she is going to do. She should elicit history of any drug reaction before.
- For the irrigation purpose, either a bottle with two glass tubes introduced through the cork, an undine, single bulb irrigator or a 20 cc syringe is used. For home use, "eye cup" is employed. The cup is filled with clean water (or saline); the patient bends over it, keeps the eye over the fluid in the cup and then blinks into the solution.
- She must check the label on the container. Fluid from container which has no label on it should never be used. It is preferable that the solution is warmed to body temperature. The solution is poured on the back of the nurse's hand to check its temperature. It should not be hot.
- The patient is asked to lie down on the couch. The head is minimally tilted to the side of the eye to be washed. The patient is draped up to the neck so that inadvertently his dress is not drenched. Cotton plug is put inside the ipsilateral ear. In very agitated patient a drop of local anaesthetic may be used. But it is better to avoid this because local anaesthetic itself causes irritation of the eye. The area surrounding the lids is cleaned. The nurse puts on disposable gloves.
- The irrigator is kept about 2 inches above the eye. The lids are kept apart by the nurse with her fingers. The fluid stream is to fall at the medial canthus (angle of eye). The stream should be directed away from the nose so that the fluid washes the eye and flows out over the temple. The fluid should not fall on the cornea directly.
- Tip of the irrigator should not touch the lids or eyelashes.
- Instead of this single stage irrigation method, the washing can be done in stages. The lower lid is drawn down so that

the inferior portion (fornix) of the conjunctiva is washed. The eye ball should not be pressed. The upper lid is everted and the conjunctiva on the back of the upper lid is washed. The eversion of upper lid may be a bit painful in many patients. If needed a drop of anesthetic drops may be applied in the eye. But it is better to avoid this.

- The irrigation returns are caught in a kidney tray. Irrigation is done till the fluid from the eye is clean or till the fluid in the bulb syringe is exhausted. Patient may be asked to blink in between the irrigation. This moves pus from upper to lower conjunctiva.
- At the end, the remaining pus is wiped off carefully with sterile cotton. It must be done from medial canthus outwards. The cornea should not be scratched. The excess fluid on the face is wiped out with clean towel. The ear plug is removed. The recommended drug is instilled.
- Assess the patient for a few minutes before he goes away.
- All relevant details are documented including any reaction patient might have had.

PATCHING OF EYE

Equipment needed
1. Eye pad (patch)
2. Sterile tray with cotton balls
3. Eye bandage/paper plaster
4. Large scissors
5. Medicines

In many places *'patch'* for the eye is known as 'pad'. It is of about 1" thick with cotton kept between gauze. It is cut into a square of about 2". It can be trimmed at one corner so that it conforms to the shape of orbital area to accommodate the nasal region (Fig. 3.2). For pressure bandage, more than one pad (patch) is used. The first pad is folded into half lengthwise and is kept on the closed eyelids. The second unfolded pad is kept over it. In some centers, the patch consists of gauze only without any cotton. This might not be very effective if the discharge from eye is much. Patient is asked to close BOTH the eyes before patching.

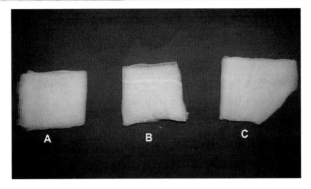

Figure 3.2: The eye pads (patch). It can be of cotton with gauze on both sides (A) or can be of gauze only (B). For pressure bandage, one corner of pad is snipped off (C)

The patch is *held* in place by many ways:

1. By a bandage which has four tails. One pair of tails is tied over the head and the other pair under the cheek. This method is employed if both the eyes are to be covered (Fig. 3.3).
2. By a bandage which has no tail. This is for covering only one eye. A 24" long and 2" broad cloth is taken and an opening is

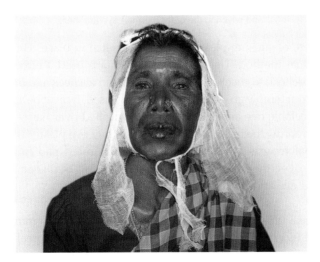

Figure 3.3: Four tail bandage. The upper and lower tails are already tied. After placing the pads (patches) over the eyes, the two tails on the sides will be brought in front and tied over the pads. This is mostly used for bandaging both the eyes

made at the junction of its 2/3rd and 1/3rd. The hole is for ipsilateral ear lobe. On the other side the bandage is taken over the parietal prominence and tied (Fig. 3.4). With the latter method there is a possibility that the contralateral eye may be covered by the bandage or the bandage itself may slip down from the parietal prominence and get loosened.

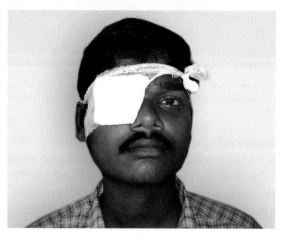

Figure 3.4: Single eye bandage. Chances of loosening of the bandage and covering the other (normal) eye are there

3. Use of sticking plaster to keep the patch in place. This is the ideal method. Usually two plasters are used – either from forehead to cheek, or one from forehead to cheek and the other from temple area to nose. If plaster is used, it must be an easily peelable one and it should not be applied over hair – that of eyebrow, beard or hair over head. Paper eye plaster is ideal.

If patching is needed and at the same time if pad cannot be placed over the eye, then a fenestrated *shield* is placed on the affected eye and patched.

Nowadays the indications and uses of eye pad are coming down. In corneal ulcer, except where "support" is needed (as in cases of corneal ulcer threatening perforation or perforated corneal ulcer), patching is not done. This facilitates the hourly drops application.

Patching after cataract surgery (especially day surgery case) is a subject for controversy. Patching with local antibiotics protects the operated eye and reduces the risk of endophthalmitis. If patching is not used after cataract surgery, *"instant vision"* is obtained giving assurance to patient. But this vision is a blurred one during the first eight hours (this must be explained to patient) and patient may become apprehensive. In "instant vision" method there may be pain and discomfort due to dryness of eye. Both methods are acceptable. Patient's choice must be given importance.

It is preferable to patch cases that have undergone pterygium and sac surgeries.

COMPRESSES

1. *Hot compress*—By hot compress it is meant warm compress. The heat relieves pain and increases circulation. This results in reducing tension in the eye. This is valuable for any deep seated as well as for superficial inflammations of the eye.
   - *A towel is put over the patient's chest*
   - *A gauze or a clean towel is dipped in water which is at a temperature of 120° F. This is placed over the closed lids.*
   - The compress is kept for one minute and changed.
   - This is done for ten changes and repeated once in four hours
   - Every time the lids should be dried with cotton
   - Fresh basin of warm water and a new set of compresses should be used for the other eye, if there is a need for the second eye.

2. *Cold compress*—This causes constriction of small vessels thereby reducing the secretion and pain. This is not useful for deep-seated conditions such as iritis.
   - *A towel is put over the patient's chest*
   - *A gauze or a clean towel kept over a block of ice is taken. This is placed over the closed lids.*
   - The compress is kept for one minute and changed.
   - This is done for ten changes and repeated once in four hours.
   - Every time the lids should be dried with cotton.
   - New set of compresses should be used for the other eye, if there is a need to apply cold compress to the other eye.

TONOMETRY

It is a procedure by which the intraocular pressure (IOP) is measured with the help of instruments. Without instruments the ocular pressure can be approximately checked by using fingers (Fig. 3.5). This needs experience by the examiner. Instruments that are used to measure the IOP are called *tonometers*. These tonometers can either be those which touch the cornea while measuring the intraocular pressure or those which do not touch the cornea when the measurement is being taken.

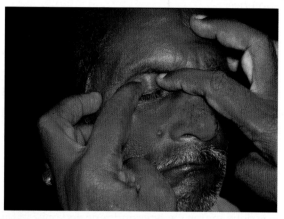

Figure 3.5: Digital tonometry. Method of finding out whether the ocular pressure is raised or not. One finger is kept steady. Minimal pressure is given with the other finger and the fluctuation of the eyeball that is felt by the first finger gives an idea of the intraocular pressure

The most popular models amongst those which touch the cornea are Schiotz tonometer and Goldmann applanation tonometer. The latter is more accurate; but needs an apparatus called slit lamp. Whichever tonometer is used, proper sterilisation is a must.

Schiotz tonometer is a tonometer which depresses the cornea to measure the intraocular pressure. The reading is given on an arched scale over which a pointer moves (Figures 3.6 and 3.7). The range of this pointer movement depends upon the intraocular pressure. The reading on the scale is noted and the intraocular pressure is read out from a standard chart. The weight of the tonometer plunger can be increased (which is needed if the reading is less than 4 on the arched scale) by adding weights. The normal intraocular pressure is from 8.0 to 21.0 mm of Hg.

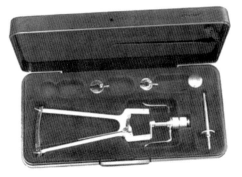

Figure 3.6: Schiotz tonometer. This is used for measuring intraocular pressure

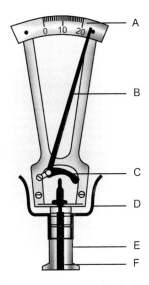

Figure 3.7: Parts of Schiotz tonometer. A – Scale. B – Indicator needle.
C – Hammer. D – Handle. E – Cylinder. F – Plunger

Equipment needed–
1. Schiotz tonometer in a sterile tray
2. Tetracaine (2%) drops
3. Sterile, wet cotton balls
4. Antibiotic eye drops

The Schiotz *tonometer* must be kept in a sterile container during the out patient hours. The container box of the tonometer is usually not sterile. So, it is preferable that, in the morning, the tonometer is taken out of the box, the accuracy of the instrument checked with the test base in the box and then sterilised. The tonometer is disassembled. The barrel cleaned with a pipe cleaner soaked in alcohol and dried. The plunger is cleaned with alcohol soaked cotton swab and allowed to dry. Ether should not be used. The instrument is re-assembled. After this it can be kept in a sterile container like a tray for the day's office work. In between cases it is enough if the foot plate is cleaned with alcohol soaked cotton swab. Some recommend simple washing of the plunger end and the foot plate with sterile water. At the end of the day, the instrument must be dismantled, thoroughly cleaned with wet cotton and kept in the container box.

Usually the *tonometry* (the procedure of measuring the intraocular pressure) with Schiotz tonometer is done by the technician. But some times, especially in camps and survey, the staff nurse may be required to perform tonometry.

- Before doing tonometry, it is ideal to clean the lids of all dirt with sterile, wet cotton.
- Locally 2% proparacaine or tetracaine (one drop) is applied in each eye. The points to remember while applying anaesthetic drop to eye are – 1) There is some amount of irritation (or even pain) in the eye on instillation of anaesthetic drops. Patient must be warned about this; otherwise patient is bound to think that a wrong drug has been applied. 2) Frequent blinking helps in overcoming this irritation. 3) It is ideal to instill for the second time after a minute (the irritation is less during this second instillation). 4) Tonometry must be done two minutes after the first (or second) instillation. The drug would have started acting by then.
- It is better to measure the left eye first. Left eye lids are kept apart with the fingers of examiner's left hand. She holds the tonometer with the thumb and forefinger of right hand and pulls up the upper lid of patient's right eye with the ring and little fingers of her own right hand. This helps the other (right) eye open during tonometry of left eye. If the other eye is not kept open, patient may get agitated when the tonometer approaches the eye to be measured (which blocks the vision).

- The patient is asked to look straight ahead. Patient should not attempt to close the eyes.
- The tonometer should not be pressed hard on the cornea. If the reading is less than 4, additional weights are added to the plunger (Fig. 3.8).

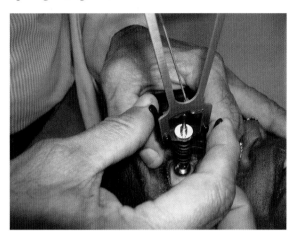

Figure 3.8: Tonometry. Measuring intraocular pressure (tonometry) with Schiotz tonometer

- At the end of tonometry, antibiotic drops are applied in the eyes.
- The patient must be warned that the eye will be anaesthetic for about 30 minutes and must be cautioned against foreign body falling into his eyes.
- Schiotz tonometer is easy to use and carry, and does not require much practice or costly equipment. But it can give wrong readings if the sclera is not having normal rigidity. Carelessness or wrong methodology also can result in false values.

Tonometry with *applanation tonometer* is the duty of ophthalmologist.

The applanation tonometer (popular model is Goldmann) has a double prism head attached by a rod to the housing which delivers a measured force (Fig. 3.9). Slit lamp is needed to use these tonometers. Tonometry with applanation tonometer gives correct value (Fig. 3.10).

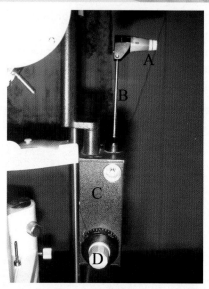

Figure 3.9: Applanation tonometer (Goldmann). The intraocular pressure can be measured more accurately with this instrument. A – Double prism. B – Rod. C – Housing. D – Force adjustment knob

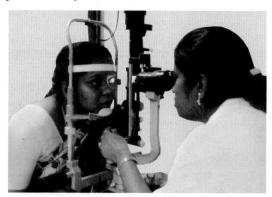

Figure 3.10: Tonometry. Intraocular pressure measurement with Goldmann applanation tonometer

Equipment needed –
1. Slit lamp
2. Applanation tonometer
3. Freshly prepared sterile fluorescein (2%) eye drops
4. Tetracaine (2%) drops

5. Antibiotic eye drops
6. Sterile cotton balls – both dry and moist
7. Kidney tray
   • The nurse must clean the slit lamp in the morning. The prism of the tonometer must be cleaned and kept sterile. Freshly prepared sterile, 2% fluorescein and 2% lignocaine drops must be kept ready along with sterile cotton balls. It is the duty of nurse to explain to the patient the procedure and infuse courage into him.
   • If the patient leaves the outpatient immediately after tonometry, he must be warned that the eye will be anaesthetic for another 30 minutes.

NASOLACRYMAL PASSAGE INVESTIGATIONS

Equipment needed
1. 2 cc syringe with blunted 22 G needle which is bent 5 mm from the blunt tip.
2. Nettleship punctum dilator (various sizes).
3. Bowman's lacrymal probe(various sizes).
4. Fluorescein (2%) mixed in saline.
5. Lignocaine (2%) eye drops.
6. Kidney tray.
7. Sterile cotton balls.
8. Antibiotic drops.
   The investigation of nasolacrymal passage may stop with canaliculus or may go up to nasolacrymal duct for detecting any nasolacrymal duct block.
   • Dilatation of punctum is needed first. Basic knowledge of anatomy is a must while carrying out this investigation. The punctum is situated about 6 mm from the medial canthus in both upper and lower lids. From punctum the canaliculus goes straight down (lower lid) or up (in upper lid) before turning almost 90° inwards to run upto Lacrymal sac. The two canaliculi may open separately into sac or join together as common canaliculus and open into sac. Dilatation must be done for punctum only. The punctum dilator should not be used beyond the punctum.

- Nurse should explain to the patient what is going to be done. She must tell him that drug may come into his oropharynx.
- Local anaesthetic agent is a must (precautions mentioned earlier are followed). It should be instilled at least thrice at one minute interval.
- The lid is cleaned of any pus and dirt that might be present.
- The lower lid is pulled down. By rotatory movement with a sterile Nettleship punctum dilator the punctum is dilated. This step is enough to cure certain conditions of punctum such as congenital atresia of punctum.
- If further study of lacrymal passage is needed, either probing with a lacrymal probe or syringing is resorted to.
- For *probing*, after dilating punctum (Fig. 3.11), a lacrymal probe (Bowman's) is passed vertically for 2 mm, then turned inwards for 90° and passed till it hitches against the lacrymal bone. This means the tip is in lacrymal sac. If probing of nasolacrymal duct is required, the probe is turned down by 90° and passed further. This procedure helps in - 1) finding the site of obstruction and 2) relieving the obstruction.

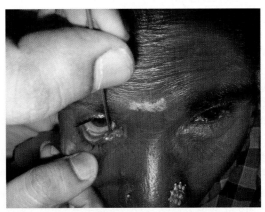

Figure 3.11: Probing of lacrymal passage. This is done after local application of anaesthetic drops

- Many a time the patency of lacrymal passage is checked by *Jones dye test I* – One drop of 2% fluorescein is instilled into the conjunctival sac (eye) and patient is asked to blink a few times. The opposite nostril is closed with finger pressure on ala of nose.

Cotton is placed at the ipsilateral nostril opening and the patient is asked to blow the nose. If the nasolacrymal passage is patent, the cotton is stained with fluorescein (green).

- In case the above test (which is a physiological one) is negative, *syringe test (Jones dye test II)* is carried out – A 2 CC syringe filled with saline is taken in which 3 drops of 2% fluorescein is added. A 24 G needle with the bevel snipped off and bent about 5 mm from the tip is attached to the syringe.
- Local anaesthetic drops are instilled. Before syringing the patient must be told that some fluid may flow into his throat. If this caution is not given, some patients tend to react violently when he gets the syringed fluid in his throat. The needle is gently introduced into the vertical portion of canaliculus (usually the lower one) and the solution injected (Fig. 3.12). The needle introduction must be gentle. If a false passage is created, then the procedure is abandoned or it is done through the other punctum (upper).

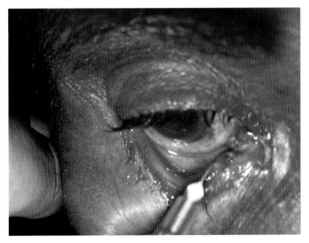

Figure 3.12: Syringing. The needle (blunted) tip need not go beyond the vertical portion of canaliculus

- If the nasolacrymal duct is patent – 1) The patient himself will tell that the fluid has come into his nasopharynx, or 2) if the patient is asked to spit, the spittoon will be stained greenish. During probing and syringing the patient should not move the head.

- If the passage is not patent, the fluid regurgitates. The nurse must observe the puncta for—
  a. The regurgitating may occur immediately and through the same punctum. This means that there is canalicular obstruction and that the common canaliculus is absent.
  b. The regurgitation may happen almost immediately through the other (upper) punctum. This means that the common canaliculus is present and that the obstruction is beyond this but proximal to sac.
  c. The regurgitation may occur after injecting some amount of fluid (the obstruction is beyond the sac.) The nature of regurgitant should be observed – whether it contains pus or mucous.

As mentioned before, the patient must be cautioned about his eyes being without sensation for about 30 minutes after the test.

The nasolacrymal passage can be outlined and site of block visualised by *dacryocystogram.* In this procedue an oil soluble dye is injected into the lacrymal passage and X' ray taken.

The syringing test and the other investigations mentioned above should never be done if there is local acute inflammation or if rhinosporidium infection is suspected.

VISUAL ACUITY TEST

Both distance and near vision are to be checked. *Distance vision* is tested with Snellen's chart which has 7 lines in it (Fig. 3.13). The top most line (letter) can be read at a distance of 60 meters by a person with normal vision. A person with normal sight can read the last (seventh) line at a distance of 6 meters. The patient is kept at 6 meters (20 feet) and asked to read the chart. If he can read the seventh line, then he is said to be having 6/6 (20/20) vision, i.e. normal vision. If he can read, for example, the fourth line only from the top and not beyond, then he is said to be having a vision of 6/18 (20/60). The numeric notation used is given on the left side of chart. Many use the terms OD and OS for right eye and left eye respectively.

To find out whether a person's defective vision is due to refractive error or not, pin hole test is done. If the vision improves with pin hole, it means that the defective vision is due to refractive error.

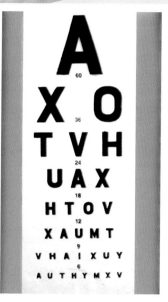

Figure 3.13: Snellen's Chart. This is used for checking the acuity of vision. Person with normal vision must be able to read the seventh line at a distance of 6 meters (20 feet). This is written as 6/6

Refractive error is checked by the procedure known as retinoscopy using trial set containing lenses of various powers (Fig. 3.14).

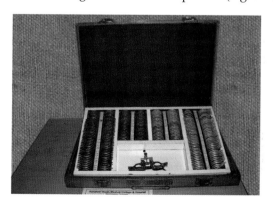

Figure 3.14: Trial set. It contains the basic lenses. With this, patients with refractive error are examined for the glasses power they need. The central four rows are cylinder lenses. The right side two rows are convex spherical lenses (+ lenses) and the left side two rows are concave spherical lenses (– lenses). The trial frame is also seen in this photo

Near vision is the ability of a person to see clearly within 30 cms (i.e. reading, etc). Here also numeric notations are used to record the vision. For example, J2 (or N6) is normal near vision. Near vision test chart is used. The illumination must be of similar intensity as patient's work area (Fig. 3.15).

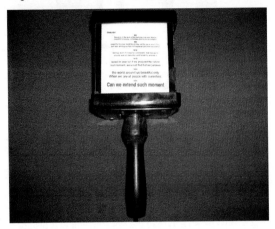

Figure 3.15: Chart used for checking near vision. It is a self illuminated one. But it is ideal to check near vision under the usual room illumination

The nurse must familiarise herself with *color vision test* with Ishihara chart (Fig. 3.16). It is used to detect red-green defect the patient may have. Each eye has to be tested separately. The colour plates are of four categories.

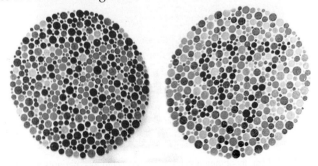

Figure 3.16: Color vision chart. These are two sample charts from Ishihara's set of colour vision charts. The number on the left side is 16 and on the right side 97 for a person with normal colour vision. A person who is colour blind for red-green will not be able to read the numbers or will read them wrongly

OTHER TESTS

There are certain other tests which are done in outpatient area. These tests are fundus study (viewing the interior of the eye) with direct or indirect *ophthalmoscope* (Figs 3.17 and 3.18). In these equipment, a beam of light is reflected through the pupil and makes it possible for the examiner to see the vitreous and retina. This procedure is known as ophthalmoscopy (Fig. 3.19). Blood vessels in retina can be seen – only site in the body where blood vessels can be directly seen. It is the duty of nurse to keep the ophthalmoscope in its proper case after use. The lenses in the direct ophthalmoscope should be cleaned (if there is a need) only by trained technician.

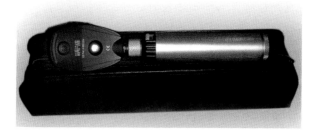

Figure 3.17: Direct ophthalmoscope. To view the fundus of eye

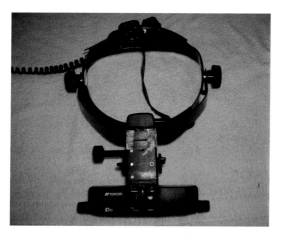

Figure 3.18: Indirect ophthalmoscope. To view the interior (fundus) of eye. With this instrument, it is possible to see the eye interior from a distance

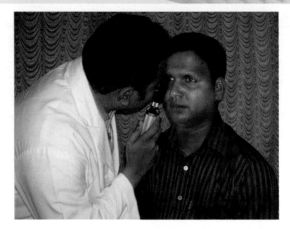

Figure 3.19: Ophthalmoscopy. The procedure of viewing the ocular fundus
with direct ophthalmoscope

Field study with dynamic or static perimeter is usually done by
trained technicians (Fig. 3.20). The extent of the field is 90° all around
with depression in the upper (because of eye brow) and the lower
inner area (because of the ala of nose). The inner one third of the
field of vision (i.e. 30°) is known as central field. The field contains
a fixation point in the middle (which corresponds to the macula)
and a blind spot (which corresponds to the optic disc) (Fig. 3.21).
The field is studied either with moving objects (kinetic perimetry)
or with stationary objects (static perimetry) (Fig. 3.22).

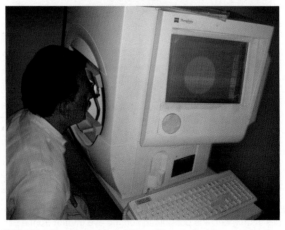

Figure 3.20: Charting the field of vision with a static (computerised) perimeter

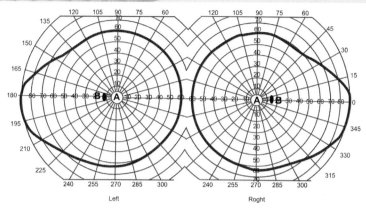

Figure 3.21: Perimeter chart used for dynamic perimeter. A – Fixation point (Corresponds to macula). B – Blind spot (Corresponds to optic disc)

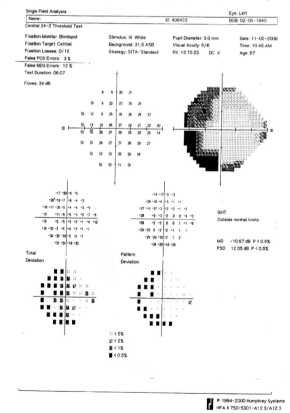

Figure 3.22: Perimeter chart of a patient taken with static perimeter

Study with biomicroscope (*slit lamp*) gives a magnified view of eye structures in front of pupil (Fig. 3.23). It is also used to check the intraocular pressure by applanation method. The fundus can also be viewed with the help of slit lamp using Hruby lens. Another examination that is possible with slit lamp is study of angle of anterior chamber. This is done with *gonioscope* (goniolens) (Fig. 3.24) and the procedure itself is known as gonioscopy (Fig. 3.25).

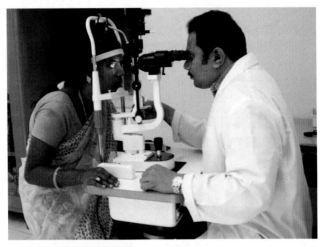

Figure 3.23: Examination of a patient with slit lamp (biomicroscope)

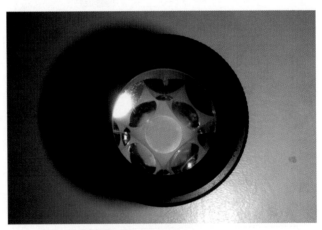

Figure 3.24: Gonio lens. This instrument is used to view the angle of anterior chamber

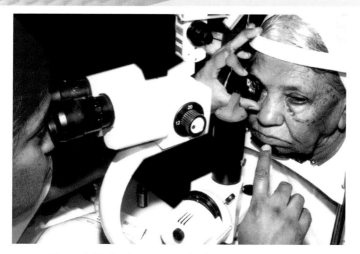

Figure 3.25: Gonioscopy examination of angle of anterior chamber using goniolens

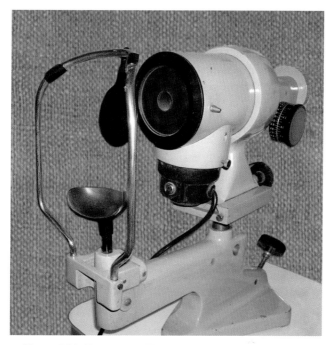

Figure 3.26: Keratometer. The corneal curvature is measured with this instrument

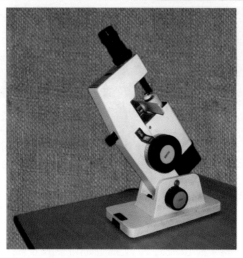

Figure 3.27: Lensmeter. This instrument is used for checking
the power of lenses in spectacles

Goniolens is a contact lens with (as in Goldmann goniolens) or without mirror (Koeppe lens) device. It is of special use in study of glaucoma cases. Since these lenses come in contact with patient's cornea, it should be properly sterilised by the nurse (See chapter 10 on "Instruments"). Other instruments used in out patient are *Keratometer* (Fig. 3.26) (to measure the corneal thickness) and *lens meter* (Fig. 3.27) (to find the power of lenses in the spectacles).

4

Anatomy of Eye and Its Adnexa

The eye ball (Fig. 4.1) is almost a sphere (ball) and has a non vascular, transparent, colorless structure in front called cornea. It is situated inside the bony orbit which is made of seven bones. The eye ball is surrounded by fatty tissue. Apart from eye ball, the bony orbit contains lacrymal gland, lacrymal sac and extra ocular muscles. The eye ball is divided into two portions – the anterior one containing cornea, iris, lens and aqueous humor (a transparent fluid). The posterior portion has vitreous, retina and choroid.

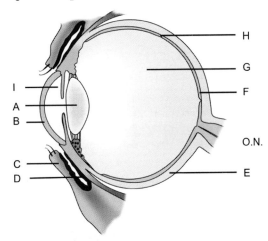

Figure 4.1: Cross section of eye. A – Lens. B – Cornea. C – Lid. D – Conjunctiva. E – Sclera. F – Choroid. G – Vitreous. H – Retina. I – Iris. O.N. – Optic nerve

Cornea is a round, transparent, colorless structure. It is 11 mm in size and is 0.5 to 1.0 mm thick. It has five layers. From before backwards they are epithelium, Bowman's membrane, stroma, Descemet's membrane and endothelium. If destroyed Bowman's membrane cannot regrow resulting in some amount of corneal opacity. Cornea is richly supplied by nerves from trigeminal nerve and is a very sensitive structure. There are no vessels in it. It has a refractive power (capacity to focus) of +43 D. Two third of the refraction (converging the outside rays of light to retina) by eye is by cornea.

Sclera occupies the remaining 4/5th of globe's circumference. It is fibrous, tough, almost non vascular, protective coat of the eye ball. It joins the cornea in front at *Limbus*. On the outside it has Tenon's capsule and bulbar conjunctiva and on the inside choroid. It is pierced by: a) apertures for ciliary vessels and nerves behind, b) apertures (near equator) for vortex veins, and c) openings (4 mm from limbus) for anterior ciliary vessels. Long ciliary nerves supply it. Actually the white of eye that is seen is the sclera (covered by almost transparent conjunctiva).

Anterior chamber is the space between cornea in front and lens-iris behind. At its periphery is its angle which is covered by sieve-like trabecular meshwork. Through this angle the aqueous humor goes out of the eye.

Uveal Tract is the vascular coat of the eye and consists of iris in front, choroid behind and ciliary body in between. In the middle of *Iris* is the pupil and just outside to it is the frill like collarette. Iris is richly supplied by blood vessels and nerves. It has two sets of muscles – dilator and constrictor muscles (of pupil). Color of "the eye" is actually the color of iris seen through the colorless, transparent cornea.

Ciliary body is the next portion of uveal tract. It is a triangular structure and contains ciliary muscles. It is also richly supplied by blood vessels. Ciliary body has two regions – posterior region which is smooth (pars plana) and anterior region which is 2 mm in breadth and has finger like ciliary processes (pars plicata). Ciliary processes are about 70 in number and are the site of aqueous production. From ciliary processes arise suspensory ligaments which suspend the lens.

The posterior portion of uveal tract is *Choroid* which is the vascular coat of eye and source of nutrition to the eye.

Arterial supply to iris and ciliary body is from long posterior and anterior ciliary arteries. Choroid derives its blood supply from short posterior ciliary arteries.

The *Posterior chamber* is between the iris in front and the ciliary body – suspensory ligaments behind. It is filled with aqueous humor.

The *Lens* is a biconvex structure hung from ciliary process by zonules behind the iris. The lens is 10 mm in size and has a capsule outside, a nucleus in the center and cortex in between (Fig. 4.2). One third of focusing of light rays from outside onto retina is by lens.

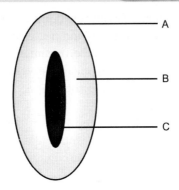

Figure 4.2: Lens. A – Capsule. B – Cortex. C – Nucleus

Retina is a transparent membrane lining the choroid and is mainly of nerve tissue. It stops short of ciliary body and this anterior limit is known as ora serrata. Retina has ten layers – outer pigment layer and inner nine neural layers. It has photoreceptors called rods and cones. The former is for night time vision and the latter is for day vision. At its posterior pole is macula. At the centre of macula is fovea centralis (Fig. 4.3). This is the point for acuity of vision and has only cones.

Medial to macula is the beginning of optic nerve which is called optic disc. This has a shallow cup. From its centre, emerges central

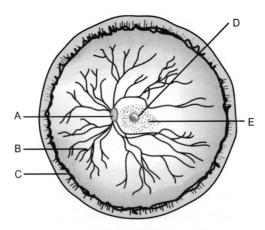

Figure 4.3: Retina (spread out). A – Optic nerve. B – Retinal vessels.
C – Ora serrata. D – Fovea centralis. E – Macula lutea

retinal artery and through this exits the central retinal vein. These vessels supply the inner layers of retina. Outer layers are nourished by choroidal vessels.

Vitreous is a transparent, gelly like mass that occupies most of the interior of the eyeball. It gives shape to the eye ball.

OCULAR ADNEXA

CONJUNCTIVA

It is almost a transparent mucous membrane lining the back of the lids (known as palpebral conjunctiva) and the front of sclera (bulbar conjunctiva). These two portions meet beneath the lids and this area of conjunctiva is known as fornix. The conjunctiva has goblet cells in it whose secretion keeps the surface of conjunctiva and cornea moist. Conjunctiva is richly supplied by nerves and blood vessels. The vessels around the cornea (anterior conjunctival vessels) are different from the blood vessels supplying other areas of conjunctiva.

Lids

The two lids – upper and lower – protect the eye from dust, foreign bodies and excess light and help in keeping the anterior surface of eye moist by spreading the tear film over it. The two lids meet at inner (medial canthus) and outer (lateral canthus) angles. The space between the open lids is known as palpebral fissure (Fig. 4.4). At the margin of the lids are fine hairs known as cilia. The lids have tarsal plates (which give shape to lids), Meibomian glands embedded in the tarsal plates, glands of Zeis and Moll which open into the base of cilia and fibers of orbicularis oculi muscle. The upper lid has, in addition, fibers of levator palpebrae superioris muscle attached to upper border of tarsal plate. The lids have skin in front and conjunctiva lining its posterior surface (Fig. 4.5). Orbicularis oculi is supplied by facial (7th cranial) nerve and the levator palpebrae superioris by oculomotor (3rd cranial) nerve.

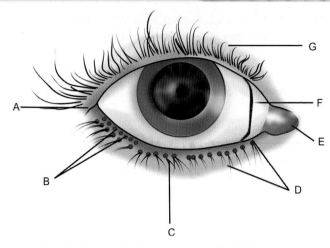

Figure 4.4: Palpebral fissure. A – Lateral canthus. B – Meibomian duct openings. C – Lower lid. D – Cilia. E – Medial canthus. F – Palpebral fissure (space between the two open lids). G – Upper lid

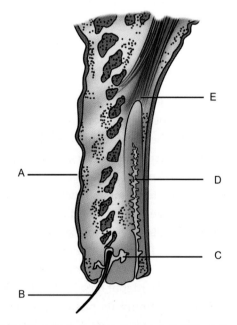

Figure 4.5: Lid (Cross section). A – Skin. B – Eye lash (Cilium). C – Glands of Zeis and Moll. D – Meibomian gland. E – Fibers of levator palpebrae superioris

Lacrymal Passage

The lacrymal gland, situated at supero lateral angle of orbit, secretes tear which is drained via lacrymal passage. This passage starts with upper and lower puncta which are situated near the medial canthus in upper and lower lids. From puncta, the canaliculi run first vertically and then turn inwards to end in the lacrymal sac. The lacrymal sac continues down as nasolacrymal duct and ends in the lower part of nasal cavity (Fig. 4.6).

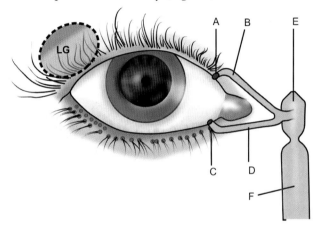

Figure 4.6: Lacrymal passage. It starts with the two puncta (one in each lid A and C). From the punctum, the canaliculus runs vertically for 1 mm, then turns inwards and runs horizontally for 7 mm (B and D). The canaliculi end in lacrymal sac (E) situated between the eye and the nose. From lacrymal sac the passage runs down as nasolacrymal duct (F) and ends in the nasal cavity. [Lacrymal gland (LG) which secretes tear is situated near the upper and outer angle of orbit]

Orbit

It is quadrilateral bony cavity at the posterior end of which is apex. The orbit contains eyeball, extra ocular muscles, fat, lacrymal gland and lacrymal sac.

Extraocular Muscles

There are six extra ocular muscles which move the eye ball. They are superior, inferior, medial and lateral recti muscles, and superior and inferior oblique muscles. Except the last one, the other five muscles are attached to eye ball in front and to apex of orbit behind. The lateral rectus is supplied by abducent (6th cranial) nerve, the superior oblique by trochlear (4th cranial) nerve and the rest of muscles by oculomotor (3rd cranial) nerve. These muscles move the eye ball in various directions. They also co-ordinate movements of both the eyes.

Visual Pathway

The route by which the stimulus from retina reaches the brain is called visual pathway. The eye nerve fibers from retina go out of the eye as optic nerve. Optic nerve enters the interior of skull and joins the nerve from the other eye at chiasma. Here the fibers of inner half of each optic nerve cross over to other side. From chiasma the fibers continue as optic tract. The optic tract ends at lateral geniculate body where the nerve fibers synapse (connect) with next nerve fibers called optic radiation. Optic radiation travels back in brain and ends at the back portion of the brain at visual cortex (Fig. 4.7).

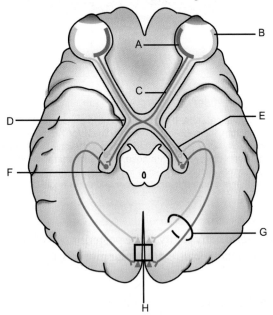

Figure 4.7: Visual pathway. It starts at retina (A and B), goes as optic nerve (C) and meets the other side eye nerve at chiasma (D). It continues further as optic tract (E) and synapses (transmits) with the next set of nerve fibers at lateral geniculate body (F). These next set of fibers continue as optic radiation (G). Finally the visual pathway ends at occipital cortex (H)

5

Physiology

Vision is possible only by focusing of light rays coming from an outside object on the retina. The focusing is by cornea and lens which converge the light rays at macula of retina. The converging of light rays takes place mainly (2/3rd) at cornea than at the lens, as is normally thought of. To facilitate the rays to reach the retina, the in between tissues (called refractive media) should be transparent – cornea, aqueous humor, lens and vitreous.

Rays from objects less than 6 meter distance from the person are diverging and so require stronger lens to focus on the retina. This increase in the power of human lens is brought about by a process called accommodation. This is brought about by the contraction of ciliary muscle (in the ciliary body). This results in the lens becoming more convex and thus become more powerful (Fig. 5.1).

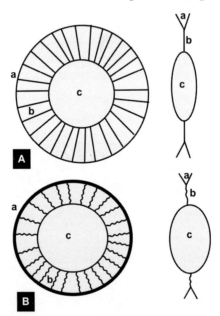

Figure 5.1: Accommodation. a – Ciliary muscle. b – Zonules. c – Lens. In the unaccommodated state (A) the zonules are tight and the lens is under traction. So the lens is less convex. During accommodation (B), the ciliary muscles contract. Due to this, the zonules are relaxed. The lens becomes more convex and the hypermetropia (+ power) increases. Small objects at or nearer to 33 cm from eye are now brought into focus

The shape of eyeball is mainly due to vitreous (a gel like structure) and to some extent by aqueous. Aqueous is secreted by ciliary processes and is poured into posterior chamber. (Posterior chamber is the space between the iris in front, and lens and suspensory ligaments behind). From here aqueous goes into anterior chamber (A/C) via the pupil (Fig. 5.2). It leaves the eye by two routes – 1) Trabecular route, which is via trabecular meshwork (TMW) situated at the angle and into Schlemm's canal. About 90% of aqueous flows through this route. 2) Uveoscleral route which is via ciliary body into suprachoroidal space. From here it is drained into general blood circulation.

Human lens is enclosed in an elastic transparent capsule to which are attached fine ligaments arising from ciliary processes. By the contraction and relaxation of ciliary muscle (in ciliary body) the shape and thickness of human lens are changed. This results in change in the power of the lens. The neural layer of retina has rods

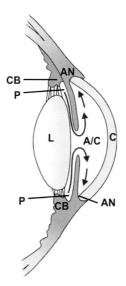

Figure 5.2: Route of aqueous in the eye. The aqueous humor is secreted by ciliary body epithelium (CB) and is poured into posterior chamber (P). From here, through the pupil, aqueous humor goes into anterior chamber (A/C) and then, via angle of anterior chamber (AN), into general circulation. (C – Cornea; L – lens)

and cones which are the receptors of light rays. The cones function for day vision. The rods are for night vision. To function during dim light, the rods require vitamin A without which the vision in dim light is markedly reduced or not possible. The nerve fibers go from retina into optic nerves. Part of the nerve crosses over at chiasma which is located under the middle part of brain. At this point the inner (nasal) fibers of optic nerve cross over to opposite side. The vision is seen by occipital cortex which is at the back of the brain.

The lacrymal (tear) gland situated at the outer and upper angle of orbit secretes the tear. Tear goes across the conjunctiva and cornea wetting them, keeping them moist, maintaining the transparency of cornea and washing off any dirt. After reaching the inner end of eye, the tear goes through the punctum, canaliculus, lacrymal sac and into the nasal cavity.

The lids open and close by the action of orbicularis oculi muscle. The upper lid is elevated by levator palpebrae muscle. The lids protect the eye from injuries, foreign bodies and excess light. They also spread the tear evenly over the conjunctiva and cornea.

6

Diseases of Eye and Its Adnexa

INTRODUCTION

The eye can be affected by infection (bacteria, fungus, virus and protozoa), allergy, immune reaction, degenerative or new growth (neoplasm). Trauma is another cause. Congenital and developmental defects are sometimes met with. Diseases of the body such as diabetes and hypertension are associated with eye problems.

While dealing with eye diseases, as with diseases elsewhere, proper history – both connected with eye and with body in general– must be taken. They are recorded in chronological (first occurred recorded first) order. Medical history includes that of diabetes, hypertension, allergy, any treatment patient is already receiving and family history.

(a) LIDS

Swellings of the lids are commonly seen in the outpatient section. Drooping, retraction, in-turning and out-turning are other lid conditions of the patients who attend the out patient section. The eyelashes may be distorted or absent.

Swellings

The conditions that frequently give rise to swellings of lids are hordeolum externum (stye), hordeolum internum and chalazion (tarsal cyst) (Figs 6.a.1 and 6.a.2). Their features and managements are given in Table 6.a.1.

Table 6.a.1: Swellings of Lids			
	H. externum	*H. internum*	*Chalazion*
Structure affected	Glands of Zeis & Moll	Meibomian (tarsal) glands	Meibomian (tarsal) glands
Etiology	Infection (especially by staphylo), refractive errors, diabetes	Infection (especially by staphylo), refractive errors, diabetes	Low grade inflammation
Pathology	Acute inflammation of the glands	Acute inflammation of the gland	Granulomatous condition

Contd...

Contd...

Onset and duration	Sudden onset with short duration	Sudden onset with short duration	Insidious onset and chronic course
Symptoms	Pain and swelling of lids	Pain and swelling of lids	Only swelling; no pain
Signs: Swelling	Nearer to skin which is adherent to it.	Deep; more towards conjunctiva, skin can be pinched over the swelling.	Deep; more towards conjunctiva, skin can be pinched over the swelling.
Tenderness	++	++	Nil
Management	Local and systemic antibiotics, analgesics, warm fomentation and drainage of pus (usually by epilation) Check for visual defect	Local and systemic antibiotics, analgesics, warm fomentation and drainage of pus (by incision and drainage) Check for defective vision.	Surgery–Incision and Curettage (I&C). Capsule should be removed. No need for antibiotics.

(If a chalazion recurs repeatedly at the same site after its surgery in an old person, one should think of cancer).

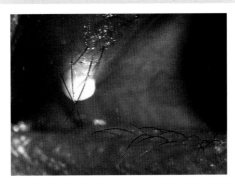

Figure 6.a.1: Hordeolum externum (Stye). The pus is pointing to the base of eyelash

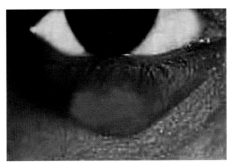

Figure 6.a.2: Chalazion

Nursing

1. In case of recurrent swelling, the nurse must insist that the patient should *check* his vision and his blood sugar (in elderly cases). The patient is liable to deny very vehemently that he is having these two problems.
2. If *hot* compress is advised, the patient must be advised to dip a cloth in WARM water and apply it over CLOSED lids. Lids do not have subcutaneous fat. So HOT compress applied over lids can cause burns.
3. If epilation is advised, it must be done after instilling local anaesthetic in the eye. The offending lash is pulled out with epilation forceps.
4. If simple epilation is done, the nurse should gently assure the patient that the eyelash may grow again.

INFLAMMATION OF LID MARGIN

It is called *blepharitis.* The two main types of blepharitis are squamous and ulcerative. In the ulcerative type, the eyelashes may be distorted or even get lost causing cosmetic disfigurement. These do not occur with squamous type. Blepharitis is *caused* by infection (especially by staphylo), eye strain and parasites such as demodex folliculorum or crab louse.

Nursing

1. The lid margin is cleaned with baby shampoo or soft soap and water. The nurse must be careful that the agent does not fall into the conjunctiva or cornea.
2. The eye ointment should be taken in the bulb of the nurse's clean finger and rubbed over the lid margin. Simple application alone without rubbing in will not be useful.

Position of Lids

The lid may be abnormally turned, drooped or retracted. Abnormal turning can be inwards (entropion) or outwards (ectropion).

Ectropion is eversion of lid margin and eyelashes away from eye.

The prominent symptom is watering from eye. Exposure keratitis (One type of corneal ulcer) and dermatitis of lids are complications that can set in.

Management is mostly surgical.

Entropion is in-turning of lids. It produces trichiasis (rubbing of eyelashes on the cornea) causing foreign body sensation, watering from eye and even corneal ulceration. The last condition may result in marked defective vision.

Management is mostly surgical correction. The nurse may be asked to pull out the eyelash (epilation) that is rubbing against the cornea.

For *nursing* instruction see under "lid swellings"

Some patients (especially ladies) may be apprehensive regarding the cosmetic 'disfigurement' the epilation might cause. The nurse should tell them that there is all possibility that the lash may grow again.

Trichiasis

Trichiasis is in-turning of eyelashes – a misdirection (Fig. 6.a.3).

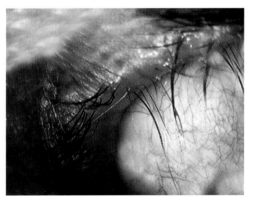

Figure 6.a.3: Trichiasis. The inturned eyelashes are rubbing against the conjunctiva (and cornea)

It is *seen in* trachoma, blepharitis and in any condition that causes entropion of lids. Local operations, severe local inflammation and burns are other causes. Only one or a few lashes may be involved, or (as in entropion) the whole row of lashes may be inturned.

Symptoms are essentially that of lashes rubbing against the cornea – foreign body sensation, pain, watering and blepharospasm (tight closure of lids). Cornea is affected by punctate (dotlike ulcers) keratitis, erosions or even by ulceration.

Management is by 1) removing the concerned cilia by epilation (may regrow), 2) destruction of hair follicle by eletrolysis or by diathermy and 3) Correction of entropion, if it is present.

Ptosis

It affects upper lid only and is mainly *due to* paralysis of levator palpebrae superioris muscle. It may be unilateral or bilateral, partial or complete, congenital or acquired.

Apart from its cosmetic problem, a complete ptosis covering the eye produces amblyopia (defective vision) in the affected eye.

Treatment is by surgery.

Nursing

1. If it is partial ptosis, the nurse must emphasize on the cosmetic problem and the possibility of being rejected for many jobs later in life.
2. If it is total (complete) ptosis, she must explain to the parents of the possibility of the involved eye of child losing most of the vision permanently and the need for early surgery.
3. The most important aspect of ptosis is that this condition is considered as luck. The nurse insists on surgery, the operation is done, something bad coincidentally happens to the family of patients and then the family turns into a sworn enemy of the nurse! The nurse should keep this in her mind.

Lagophthalmos

It is the inability to close the lids due to paralysis of facial nerve, or due to protrusion of eyeball or cornea. It can lead to exposure of cornea constantly and ulceration (exposure keratitis).

Treatment depends on the cause.

Nursing

See under "Comatose patient".

Injuries

Nurse must patch the eye immediately and inform the surgeon.

(b) LACRYMAL PASSAGE

Lacrymal sac and the nasolacrymal passage are important since they are source of problematic infection.

Lacrymal sac can be involved in inflammatory pathology and this is known as *dacryocystitis*. In this condition, the passage is blocked causing watering from eye. Dacryocystitis can be congenital, acute or chronic.

CONGENITAL DACRYOCYSTITIS

It is *due to* incomplete formation of lacrymal passage. It is prone to get infected. The parents notice watering from eye one month after birth. Cornea is of normal size and there is no other ocular problem. (Watering is also seen in ophthalmia neonatorum and buphthalmos. In ophthalmia neonatorum, watering from eye occurs within 15 days of birth. In buphthalmos, watering from eye is met with one month or more after birth. This is an important differentiating symptom that should be kept in mind by the nurse).

The *management* is by pressure over sac to empty its content and application of antibiotic drops to eye (massage treatment). This should be done three times a day and continued for at least six months before giving up. Probing the nasolacrymal passage is a one-time cure. This and syringing with antibiotic (which is also effective) need anaesthetizing the newborn. Some parents may not agree to this. If all fail, dacryocystorhinostomy (DCR) is done.

Nursing

1. She must emphasise the importance of patience while carrying out massage treatment for congenital dacryocystitis.
2. If parents are not willing for such a long treatment period, she should convince them for a short anaesthesia that is needed for probing or syringing. She must emphasise that it is safe and is one time quick cure. Even then some parents may not agree to this also.

3. The nurse must emphatically tell the parents the danger to cornea by the sac disease.
4. For massage treatment, she must teach the parents where exactly to press for emptying the lacrymal sac. She must also teach the parents how to apply eyedrops. The fingernails of the person applying drops must be trimmed.

CHRONIC DACRYOCYSTITIS

It is common in aged ladies and in poor people. It is *caused by* obstruction to nasolacrymal.

The main *complaint* is watering from eye. Swelling over sac region is seen (Fig. 6.b.1). Pressure over it results in regurgitation of pus via canaliculus and punctum. Probing reveals the site of obstruction in some cases. If entry and exit of sac both are blocked, the secretion accumulates inside sac resulting in considerable swelling. Dacryocystography with oil soluble radio-opaque dye shows the site of obstruction.

It can lead onto ulceration of cornea, acute dacryocystitis and chronic conjunctivitis. Intraocular surgery in an eye with chronic

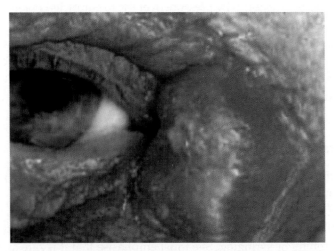

Figure 6.b.1: Chronic dacryocystitis

dacryocystitis on the same side must be undertaken only after dealing with the sac pathology.

Management is by evacuation of sac by pressure and local application of antibiotics in the eye. This may succeed. Repeated syringing with antibiotics or probing may result in cure in some cases. If these fail, either excision of sac (DCT) or DCR is done.

DCT is done in elderly and in chronic dacryocystitis with ipsilateral corneal ulcer or impending intraocular surgery. DCR is the surgery of choice in young patients.

Nursing

See under "Investigations" and "Major surgeries".

ACUTE DACRYOCYSTITIS

A chronic dacryocystitis may get infected resulting in acute dacryocystitis. The *features* are reddened skin over sac, pain, swelling over sac region and some regurgitation via punctum on pressure over sac (if pressure application is possible). There is tenderness if sac region is pressed. Abscess may form.

Management is by local and systemic antibiotics, and analgesics. If there is abscess, it should be drained. The condition resolves; but may result in chronic dacryocystitis.

Nursing

1. Warm fomentation is needed. *Hot* compress should be avoided.

Remember—No need for antibiotics for chronic dacryocystitis; but local investigations are needed. For acute dacryocystitis, no local investigation; but antibiotic is needed and is a must.

WATERING FROM EYE

It can be epiphora (Normal tear secretion; but poor drainage) or hypersecretion (Normal lacrymal passage; but excess tear production)

Epiphora is *due to* obstruction to nasolacrymal passage.

Hypersecretory type is due to lacrymal gland disease, trichiasis, foreign body of conjunctiva or cornea, conjunctivitis, scleritis, inflammation of iris and ciliary body, glaucoma, and psychogenic factors.

Constant wetting of lower lid due to epiphora may produce skin excoriation, scarring and ectropion – the last condition worsens the watering from eye and leads to a vicious circle.

Before *treatment* is undertaken, the lacrymal passage should be checked for any obstruction. Treatment is directed mostly towards the causative factor. If this does not relieve watering, DCR is done for obstructive type when the problem is in nasolacrymal passage.

Nursing

It is mostly in assessing the patency of lacrymal passage and teaching the patient how to instil eyedrops.

DRY EYE

Etiology

It may be due to deficiency of tear film. But the secretion of glands of conjunctiva is more important than tear secretion. Most important conditions are Vitamin A deficiency, trachoma, conjunctival scarring and improper lid closure.

Features

Symptoms: Burning of eyes and foreign body sensation, itching and dry feeling. Dry eye is diagnosed by carrying out various tests.

Management

1. Management of cause, if possible. It is mainly symptomatic.
2. Preservation of any tear that may be present.
3. Use of tear substitutes.

(c) CONJUNCTIVA

Conjunctival diseases are the common cases that are seen in eye out-patient department. Acute catarrhal conjunctivitis (ACCO), spring catarrh, trachoma, phlycten, pterygium and Bitot's spots are some of the cases that attend frequently.

A basic knowledge of conjunctival diseases is a must for nurses since these diseases are seen so apparent and alarm the patients very much.

While examining, eversion of upper lid must be done. Dryness, scarring, adhesion, swelling, congestion and discolouration are some of the important findings.

Conjunctivitis is inflammation of conjunctiva due to any cause. It can be infective or allergic.

In conjunctivitis, the *secretion* may be serous, mucopurulent or purulent. The *symptoms* range from foreign body sensation to severe pain in eye.

Infective conjunctivitis may be acute or chronic. The former is mainly grouped into catarrhal (mucopurulent), purulent and membranous.

The infective agents come a) from outside by air, dust, water or fomites, b) from surrounding structures such as lids and sac, or c) very rarely, via blood stream.

ACUTE CATARRHAL CONJUNCTIVITIS (ACCO)

It usually has mucopurulent discharge. It is *caused* by bacteria and rarely by virus (such as that of measles). The bacteria that usually infect are Koch-Weeks, *Staphylococcus and Streptococcus*.

Patient *complains* of foreign body sensation ("sand in the eye" feeling), sticking of lids together when getting up from sleep and discharge near canthi and over lid margin. He may give history of seeing halos. One or both eyes are involved.

The eye shows redness of conjunctiva which is more at fornix and sticking of eyelashes together (Fig. 6.c.1). Discharge is seen near medial canthus. In viral conjunctivitis the signs are less severe and the discharge is mostly watery (this condition is known as "Madras eye"). Cornea may be involved.

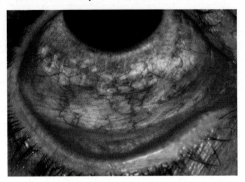

Figure 6.c.1: Acute catarrhal conjunctivitis

Management includes *prevention* of spread to other eye (in unilateral case) and to other members of family. Antibiotic drops are instilled into the unaffected eye also. The patient is isolated and other family members should use local antibiotics as preventive method.

Curative methods include washing the eye with normal saline either with a cup or with an undine (Fig. 6.c.2) (This washes away discharge and organisms). Antibiotic drops are used locally. Mostly gentamicin, framycetin or ciprofloxacin is used. Ointment is applied before patient goes to sleep to prevent gluing of lids together when the patient gets up from sleep.

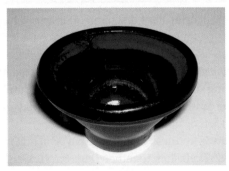

Figure 6.c.2: The cup that can be used to wash the eye at home by the patient

Nursing

1. Proper irrigation is important (See under "Procedures")
2. Drugs must be applied in the eye. Nurse must teach the patient how to apply drops to eye at home and the need for cleanliness before and after such application.
3. She must tell the patient that antibiotic drops must be applied in unaffected eye also (4 times/day) in unilateral cases.
4. She must instruct the patient not to use cortisone eye drops locally or to bandage the eye with eye pad. He can use naphazoline eye drops for relief.
5. If penicillin drops are used locally, the nurse must know how to prepare 10,000 units/ml drops.
6. She must instruct the patient to keep himself "isolated" from others at home so that the conjunctivitis does not spread to others.
7. She herself should be careful not to get infected. Washing her hands before and after dealing with the patient is important.

PURULENT TYPE

This occurs in newborn (ophthalmia neonatorum) or in adults (adult blenorrhoea).

Ophthalmia neonatorum is *due to N. gonorrhoea, staphylococcus, pneumococcus, streptococcus* (all bacteria) and virus. Latent period depends upon the causative organism. It is from three days (*staphylococcus*) to two weeks (virus). In newborn, infection sets in the eye before birth (due to premature rupture of membrane), during birth (if eyes are open before birth and birth canal is infected) or after birth (from fomites and fingers).

In the beginning the lids are swollen, conjunctiva is red and preauricular lymphnodes are inflamed. Generally the baby is sick. There is watering from eyes. Tears are produced one month after birth only. Hence, any watering from eye within two weeks of birth should alert the ophthalmologist/pediatrician/nurse for the possibility of ophthalmia neonatorum.

After a couple of days, pus *runs down* the cheek and other signs subside (Fig. 6.c.3). If untreated, the healing sets in with complications.

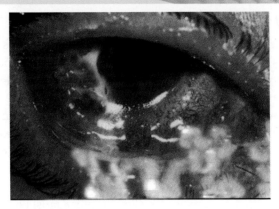

Figure 6.c.3: Purulent conjunctivitis. Pus is produced in plenty and the conjunctiva is congested

Complications are very dangerous. Cornea is easily involved, as newborn cornea is more prone for getting infected. The resultant corneal ulcer may lead to loss of eye and the sight. Xerosis (dryness of eyes) and symblepharon (gluing of conjunctiva together) are other complications.

Adult type is almost the same as that of newborn except for the mode of infection. There is more systemic involvement and systemic therapy is also more relied upon.

Management in newborn includes prevention – proper antenatal check up, and cleanliness before, during and after delivery. In suspected case, silver nitrate 1% drops are used (one drop once in each eye; Crede's method). Locally erythromycin also can be used.

Once the disease has set in, management is by frequent instillation of penicillin drops, ofloxacin, bacitracin, ciprofloxacin, tobramycin or moxifloxacin. Penicillin drops (10,000 units/cc) is instilled once a minute for 5 minutes, once in 5 minutes for 30 minutes, half hourly for two hours and then second hourly for two days (Sorsby method). While applying drops, cornea should not be scratched. If there is response, it will be obvious by the end of two hours. Pus need not be cleaned. Since penicillin resistant organisms are appearing, systemic cefotaxime or norfloxacin is used. In adults, one injection of 1 gm of cefotaxime or norfloxacin 1 gm for 5 days is effective. Corneal problem must be adequately dealt with. Chlamydial infection responds well to tetracycline.

Nursing

This is one of the few eye conditions in which a nurse can prevent blindness by her sincere attention and health education.

In this one condition ophthalmologist, obstetrician and pediatrician have a role to play.

1. The nurse should insist on pregnant mothers for the importance of proper antenatal check up.
2. Absolute cleanliness and asepsis must be observed during and after delivery.
3. If there is a suspicion that the eyes have already got infected, local antibiotic or silver nitrate must be used. Silver nitrate should NOT be instilled in the eye. It must be taken in a cotton spud, painted over the conjunctiva and the eschar (film) that forms removed. This drug should not touch the cornea.
4. The nurse should know how to prepare 10,000 units/cc of penicillin.
5. She MUST stay with the child for 2 hours and instil the drops.

MEMBRANOUS CONJUNCTIVITIS

It is *characterised* by membrane formation over palpebral *conjunctiva*. C. diphtheriae is the most feared bacteria. Others are *staphylococcus, streptococcus, N. gonorrhoeae and virus*. Most important source of the organisms is nasal cavity. Burns – either chemical or thermal, also produce membrane.

The reaction may range from minimal lid swelling, serous discharge and peelable membrane over palpebral conjunctiva (mild cases, *pseudomembranous type*) to severe edema of lids, edema with congestion of conjunctiva, chemosis and membrane (Fig. 6.c.4). This membrane is firmly adherent to conjunctiva and, when peeled, leaves behind bleeding points (*true membranous type*).

Complications are symblepharon, xerosis and trichiasis (in turning of eyelashes). More important is corneal ulcer.

During *treatment,* one should not try to peel the membrane. If this is done, the small conjunctival vessels are torn. If the condition is due to C. diphtheriae, the exotoxin of the bacteria might gain

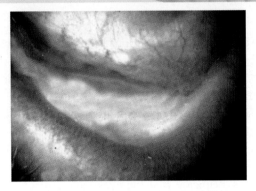

Figure 6.c.4: Membranous conjunctivitis

access to circulation and affect the heart and kidney. Starting the therapy should not wait for microbiological report.

All cases of infective membranous conjunctivitis must be considered and treated as diphtheritic unless otherwise proven by bacteriological study. Local (10,000 units per cc every 30 minutes) and systemic penicillin, and local hourly and systemic antidiphtheritic serum (20,000 units every 12 hours) are administered. All cases of infective membranous conjunctivitis, especially if diphtheritic, should be immediately referred to a pediatrician.

Nursing

1. Nurse must consider all cases of membranous conjunctivitis as diphtheritic unless the doctor says that it is not.
2. It is her duty to warn the parents and send the patient to a pediatrician without delay.
3. The nurse must tell the parents that the child must not come into connect with other children till the condition clears up.
4. If it is proven that the cause is diphtheritic, she must caution the parents about the ill effects of diphtheria, especially on the heart.
5. She herself must be careful while handling such cases.

ANGULAR CONJUNCTIVITIS

It is a chronic conjunctivitis *caused by* the bacteria, *M. lacunata* and rarely by *staphylococcus*. It is also seen in riboflavin deficiency.

There are excoriations of skin of lids and localized congestion of conjunctiva near canthi. *Symptom* (discomfort) is minimal. Blepharitis and rarely marginal or central corneal ulcer with or without hypopyon (pus in anterior chamber) are seen in long-standing cases.

Treatment is started with zinc eyedrops, which neutralizes the proteolytic enzyme produced by the organism (which causes the skin excoriation). After this, local tetracycline ointment is used which is effective against the bacteria.

Riboflavin (10 mg per day) is also given.

TRACHOMA

It is a chronic conjunctivitis *caused* by Chlamydazoa trachomatis. It is known from ancient times and is common in Mediterranean countries, Central Asia, South America and North India. It is said to be prevalent amongst Muslims and economically backward society. Flies, fingers and fomites transmit it.

Features—Conjunctiva shows redness, follicles (small, grain like lesions) and finally scarring. Follicles are seen in fornix, palpebral conjunctiva and, sometimes, over bulbar conjunctiva (Fig. 6.c.5). Scarring starts in upper palpebral conjunctiva. Later the whole conjunctiva turns into leather like tissue.

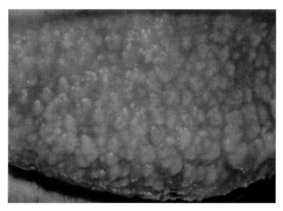

Figure 6.c.5: Case of trachoma showing follicles in conjunctiva under the upper lid

The *corneal* epithelium is involved simultaneously with conjunctiva and shows avascular superficial spots in upper portion. Later on pannus (vessels in cornea with cells) is seen. The pannus may completely resolve (except for empty vessels) or may leave behind corneal scar.

Treatment—It was once a prolonged one with sulpha drugs. Now *orally* rifampicin, tetracycline (not for children and pregnant ladies) or erythromycin (250 mg × qid) is given for four weeks. Oral doxycycline (100 mg BID.) for 3 to 5 weeks is curative.

Locally erythromycin or tetracycline (1%) applied four times a day combined with sulfacetamide (20%) and used for six weeks give equally good result. Easier is azithromycin (1 gram) as a single dose. These drugs eliminate the causative organism as well as any secondary infection. Attention must be directed towards complications.

Nursing

1. She must insist that the patient undergoes the full course of treatment
2. She must advise that the fomites used by the patient must be separate from those of the family members till his eye condition subsides.
3. It is the duty of community health nurse to check the morbidity in her area.
4. In endemic area, massive treatment scheme must be instituted.
5. Health education must be given by the nurse.

Allergic conjunctivitis is another group, in which, vernal and phlycten are the important ones.

VERNAL CONJUNCTIVITIS

It is otherwise known as *spring catarrh* or *seasonal allergic conjunctivitis*. It is *caused by* exogenous allergen such as pollen. It is seen in young patients (5 to 15 years) and occurs mostly during summer. It may be present throughout the year. Itching is the prominent *symptom*. *"No itching no spring catarrh"* is an apt statement. Spring catarrh is present either as palpebral form, bulbar form or mixed form.

In *palpebral form* flat topped, milky white, large (5 mm) papillae are seen. They are mostly in upper palpebral conjunctiva (Fig. 6.c.6). *Bulbar form* presents as discrete, white, gelatinous thickenings at limbus. It may also be present all around limbus (Fig. 6.c.7).

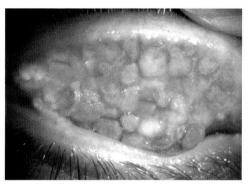

Figure 6.c.6: Case of vernal conjunctivitis affecting the upper palpebral conjunctiva. The papillae are large and have milkly white colour

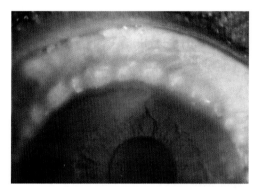

Figure 6.c.7: Vernal conjunctivitis – limbal type

Corneal involvement is rare and mostly not serious.

After a few years, the condition subsides without any ill effect.

The *secretion* in all these three types is ropy, scanty, acidic and contains plenty of eosinophils.

Management is that of symptom—local steroid, disodium cromoglycate (2%), antihistamine drops and cold compress. Olopatadine drops are used twice a day. In severe cases cyclosporine (1%) drops are used. Local naphazoline reduces itching.

Nursing

1. The first duty of the nurse is to emphasise to the parents that this condition almost never blinds the patient and that it is not a dangerous disease. She must tell them that it is a question of putting up with the itching.
2. She must caution the patient against rubbing the eyes since this may worsen the condition.
3. She must warn the parents against using cortisone for a long time, although it gives good relief.
4. She must tell the parents that this disease subsides by itself and there is NO CURE for it.

PHLYCTENULAR CONJUNCTIVITIS

In contrast to vernal conjunctivitis, this is *caused by endogenous allergen* (from inside the body of patient), which is mostly bacterial protein especially of tuberculosis. Others are *staphylococcus* and Morax-Axenfeld. Long-standing infection of tonsils or adenoids is associated with this condition.

It affects undernourished children. It is *seen in* bulbar and rarely in palpebral conjunctiva as gray, round, small nodule. Redness is seen around the nodule (Fig. 6.c.8). It may be single or multiple. Ulceration of the apex of the nodule may occur. Recurrence is common. Pure conjunctival lesion has very few symptoms such as irritation and watering. It has no complication.

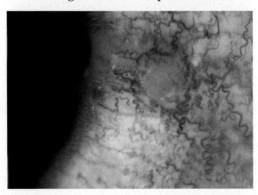

Figure 6.c.8: Phlycten affecting the conjunctiva near the limbus. There is redness around the nodule only

Limbal lesion can involve cornea resulting in phlyctenular keratitis and *fascicular ulcer*.

Treatment is by local cortisone and wearing dark glasses. Antibiotics and cycloplegics are called in if cornea is involved. Opinion differs about use of anti tuberculous treatment and desensitisation with tuberculin. Any septic focus must be taken care of. General nutrition must be attended to.

Nursing

1. The nurse should not alarm the parents by saying that the child has got tuberculosis. She must assure them that it is just a reaction to some protein in the body.
2. At the same time she must insist that the child should receive any systemic treatment the doctor might have advised.
3. She must warn the parents not to use cortisone eye drops for long.

PINGUECULA

It is seen in the aged persons as a triangular patch over palpebral conjunctiva near the limbus but not involving the cornea. It is due to dust, sunlight and wind. In some cases it may grow over cornea as pterygium.

Treatment is not needed.

PTERYGIUM

It is a subconjunctival degeneration *caused by* dust and ultraviolet rays. Sometimes pinguecula may grow as pterygium. Seen usually in persons above the age of 50 in both genders, its main *symptom* is *cosmetic* followed by *defective vision*.

It is a triangular growth partly over cornea and partly over conjunctiva. It has three *parts* – head or apex over cornea, neck at limbus and the larger portion, the body in conjunctiva. It may be fleshy or thin. It is mostly seen over inner side of cornea (Fig. 6.c.9). It has to be differentiated from pinguecula (latter does not encroach onto cornea) and pseudopterygium.

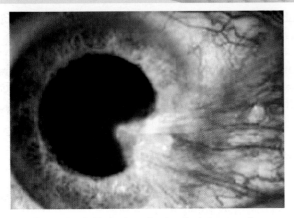

Figure 6.c.9: Pterygium. Conjunctival degeneration
which grows over cornea like a triangle

Management is a) by releasing the head and body of pterygium and excising them, or b) by implanting the released head under the conjunctiva, or c) after excision, covering the conjunctival defect with mucosal graft. Pterygium is well-known to recur after surgery. In such a case, locally Mitomycin C drops, thiotepa (1: 2000) or beta radiation (1500 rads) is used after surgery.

If the pterygium is extensive and encroaching onto the pupillary area, then a lamellar grafting is done after freeing the pterygium.

Nursing

(See under "Minor operations")

Patient must be warned about the possibility of recurrence after operation.

BITOT'S SPOTS

Bitot's spots are associated with conjunctival dryness (xerosis).

It is a manifestation of Vitamin A deficiency. If the deficiency is not corrected, it may lead to corneal ulceration resulting in keratomalacia (corneal ulcer) and blindness in children.

Bitot's spots are seen temporal (outside) to cornea as triangular aggregation of silvery white flakes with the base of triangle towards cornea (Fig. 6.c.10). They may have foamy nature. Conjunctiva is dry and dusky.

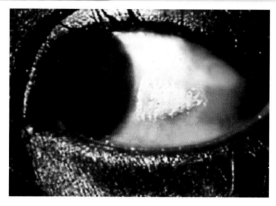

Figure 6.c.10: Bitot's spots. The conjunctiva has a dusky (dirty) colour

The patients are given 1,00,000 units of Vitamin A per day for ten days. The causative factors such as diarrhea and malnutrition must be attended to. While treating with Vitamin A the possibility of hypervitaminosis A must be kept in mind. So also the possibility of oral vitamin not being absorbed must be borne in mind. Any protein deficiency must be corrected.

Nursing

1. The nurse must have a good knowledge of diet rich in vitamin A. She must be able to advise about the diet keeping in her mind the economic status of the concerned family.
2. She must warn the parents about the child developing corneal ulcer if treatment is not properly followed.
3. She must see to it that the child is sent to the pediatrician.
4. She must have an idea about hypervitaminosis A.

SYMBLEPHARON

It is adhesion of palpebral conjunctiva to bulbar conjunctiva due to raw surfaces in them. It follows injury and burns of conjunctiva, trachoma, and dry eye. There is inability to close the eyes properly and hence problems associated with it are seen in severe cases of symblepharon.

Prevention is the best by using therapeutic bandage lens. *Treatment* is by releasing the attachment and covering the raw areas with amniotic membrane, conjunctiva or mucous membrane. A therapeutic contact lens is useful in preventing re-adhesion. Result is not always rewarding.

Nursing

If the adhesion is released and operated area left without any cover, the nurse must assist in passing a glass rod daily to prevent re-adhesion.

SUBCONJUNCTIVAL HAEMORRHAGE

It is a condition that alarms the patient. Except for this fear factor, it has no symptom by itself (Fig. 6.c.11). It is *caused by:*

1. Injury to conjunctiva or head injury involving the anterior or middle cranial fossa can cause this condition. Hemorrhage due to these two conditions should be differentiated.
2. Increase in intrathoraccic pressure as in severe cough (including whooping cough), lifting heavy weight and heavy weight over chest as in building collapse.

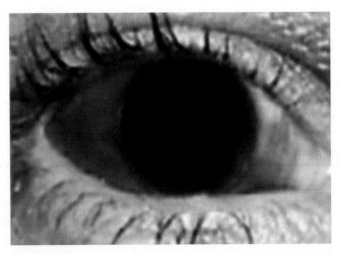

Figure 6.c.11: Subconjunctival haemorrhage due to local injury to the eye region

3. Diseases of blood vessels – Arteriosclerosis.
4. Diseases of blood – Purpura, leukaemia, aplastic anaemia.
5. Severe conjunctivitis, especially pneumococcal.
6. Systemic diseases – Hypertension, diabetes.
7. Acute fever – Malaria, diphtheria, measles.

Management is mainly that of cause. Local placebo is recommended. Patient should be reassured. Cold compress is applied.

Nursing

1. The main duty of the nurse is to assure the patient that the eye condition itself is not a big problem.
2. At the same time, she must insist that he must get himself properly treated for the causative factor.
3. She also must tell the patient that the hemorrhage may increase in size to begin with and then start disappearing.
4. She must also tell him that it will take at least 3 to 4 weeks for it to disappear and that there is no way by which it can be made to disappear early.

INJURIES

Most of the conjunctival injuries need not cause alarm. But she should be careful that the underlying sclera and other structures are not involved. Usually suturing (rarely needed) and/or patching with antibiotics are required.

(d) CORNEA

Cornea is the most important structure, as any disease in this structure can result in severe pain and defective vision. As it is so easily visible, it can alarm the patient. Corneal ulcer and scar are the common condition affecting the cornea.

Cornea is best examined by oblique illumination method or slit-lamp. Keratometry (to assess corneal curvature), pachymetry (to measure corneal thickness) and topography are some of the important specialized tests. Staining with 2% fluorescein or Bengal rose is employed in doubtful cases. Corneal surface irregularity is best checked with Placido's disc which is held in front of the cornea with source of light at the level of patient's ear on the same side.

Corneal lesions are mostly ulcer, scar, degeneration and dystrophy.

Cornea, although exposed to atmosphere and external irritants, is protected by its intact epithelium, tear (mechanical wash and by its lysozyme) and by lids. Good nutrition level of patient is equally important.

Corneal inflammation is known as *keratitis*. Based on the layer of cornea that is *first* involved, it is grouped into:

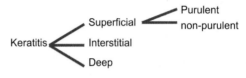

CORNEAL ULCER

It is purulent keratitis involving superficial layers of cornea to begin with. It is *caused by* bacteria, fungus and, rarely, by virus. Amongst bacteria, *C. diphtheriae* and *N. gonorrhoea* are important as they are capable of penetrating intact corneal epithelium and produce ulcer.

The *sources* of organisms are exterior (such as dust, injury), secondary (from contiguous surface such as lacrymal sac and conjunctiva) and rarely from endogenous focus (which are mostly immunological). Long time local use of steroids and antibiotics facilitates occurrence of corneal ulcer.

The *symptoms* are watering from eye, pain, defective vision, redness of eye, photophobia (sensitive to light; abolished in dark) and blepharospasm (tight closure of lids; abolished by local instillation of anaesthetic agent). Headache on the same side is present. These symptoms are sudden in onset and severe in nature.

Signs (of bacterial ulcer) are edema of lids and white opacity (the ulcer) in cornea. The opacity turns green with local instillation of fluorescein 2% drops (Fig. 6.d.1). Ciliary congestion (also known as circumcorneal congestion) is present. In this conjunctiva is dull

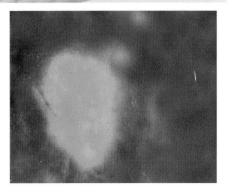

Figure 6.d.1: Corneal ulcer stained (green) with local fluorescein eye drops

red around the cornea with dilated vessels not well seen. This congestion has to be differentiated from conjunctival type of congestion of conjunctivitis in which the redness is near the fornix and the vessels are better seen.

Pus is seen in the ulcer floor and is surrounded by infiltration.

In some infections (such as pneumococcal), the bacterial toxin (and not organisms) seeps into anterior chamber, irritates iris causing pouring of cells into anterior chamber. This is *sterile* pus and settles down in anterior chamber with a horizontal upper border. It is called *hypopyon* (Fig. 6.d.2). It usually does not need draining. It is absorbed when the ulcer heals. It may cause rise in ocular pressure (controlled by oral diamox).

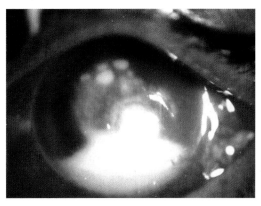

Figure 6.d.2: Hypopyon corneal ulcer. The hypopyon in this case has tented up

The pupil is small and sluggish due to iritis. Untreated, improperly treated or ineffectively treated corneal ulcer may go in for *complications*. They can occur with or without perforation of the ulcer. The infection can invade the interior of the eye ball. Cataract is sometimes seen. When the ulcer heals up, many of them result in corneal scar which is known as leucoma. In very severe cases, the cornea may perforate leading onto iris protrusion or even loss of eye.

Management of corneal ulcer follows the general surgical principles – local cleaning, control of infection, rest to inflamed parts, protection of affected area and relief from pain.

1. Before commencing treatment, *focus of infection* especially that of lacrymal sac should be excluded. Material from ulcer should be sent for microbiology study.
2. The conjunctival sac is irrigated and *cleaned* of all pus. The pus in the floor of ulcer is scraped off with fine knife. The ulcer is then cauterised with trichloracetic acid (10%) or phenol. (This should not be done in a case of perforated ulcer or for a very large ulcer with thin floor).
3. The *infection is controlled* by local and systemic use of antibiotics.
   a. Locally, antibiotic is administered in the form of drops or ointment. Hourly instillation of fortified antibiotic eyedrops has eliminated use of subconjunctival injection of antibiotic. Fortified drops are prepared by mixing in the commercial eyedrops the injection variety of the same antibiotic, or it is prepared from the systemic drug itself. Strength of certain fortified antibiotic eye drops are:
   Tobramycin (1.3%): Commercial drops + 2 ml (80 mg) of tobramycin
   Cephazolin (5%): 500 mg cephazolin + 10 ml water
   Vancomycin: 500 mg vancomycin + 10 ml sterile water
   b. Systemic antibacterial agents given must be able to cross blood-aqueous barrier since cornea is avascular. The drugs preferred for systemic administration are sulpha, chloramphenicol and cephalosporin.
4. *Rest* is needed for intraocular mobile structures – iris and ciliary body. Drugs like atropine which paralyse the iris and ciliary muscles are used once a day.

5. *Protection* is offered by bandaging the eye. Since hourly drops have to be instilled, dark glasses are advised for smaller ulcers instead of pad and bandage. Bandage contact lens can be used.
6. *Pain* is relieved by any analgesic such as paracetamol (500 mg 8 hourly) or aspirin. Warm fomentation also gives good relief.

In larger ulcer threatening perforation, ulcer with large hypopyon or in recently perforated ulcer, reduction of intraocular pressure is needed. This is achieved by oral acetazolamide tablets (250 mg 8 hourly).

Fungal corneal ulcer differs from bacterial in certain aspects. The symptoms are minimal and inflammatory signs are not much. Ulcer is typical – usually central, circular and pigmented one (Fig. 6.d.3). Slough in the ulcer is dry and raised. Hypopyon is prominent. In the diagnosis, for culture, the pus must be obtained from the depth of ulcer. In the treatment, antibiotic should never be used; only antifungal drugs such as natamycin are employed.

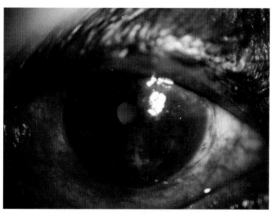

Figure 6.d.3: Fungal corneal ulcer. The pigment in the floor of the ulcer and the hypopyon are typical. The hypopyon has a horizontal upper border

Nursing

1. The foremost duty of the nurse is to encourage the patient and allay his fear.
2. Absolute cleanliness must be maintained while treating a case of corneal ulcer. The fluorescein drops must be sterile and freshly prepared.

3. She must carefully watch the corneal condition so that she can bandage the eye (instead of hourly instillation of drops) at the correct moment.
4. She must know how to prepare fortified drops.
5. For bacteriological study, pus from conjunctiva is enough. For fungal study the pus must be from the depth of ulcer. It is preferable not to apply local anaesthetic agent when taking pus for bacteriological study.

(For examination of lacrymal passage, use of eyedrops and bandaging the eye, see under "Minor procedures").

ACANTHAMOEBA KERATITIS

It is due to an amoeba, *acanthamoeba*. It invades cornea when unsterile water or saline is used while using *contact lens*.

Main *symptom* is the severe pain. Other symptoms are that of any corneal ulcer.

It starts in cornea as streaks of epithelial and subepithelial opacities. Later on it assumes a ring shape and radial *lines. Dendritic* ulcer can also occur.

Apart from treatment given to any infective corneal ulcer, locally propamidine isethionate (1%), neomycin, paramomycin or polyhexamethyle Biguanide (0.02%) is used. But very frequently corneal transplantation is required.

Nursing

1. Nurse must be aware of this condition especially if she is dealing with contact lens fixing for the patient.
2. She must definitely warn those who use contact lens about this condition; but at the same time should not alarm them.

NON-PURULENT SUPERFICIAL KERATITIS

It is seen usually with *virus* infection. The important viruses are adenovirus, herpes simplex and herpes zoster. In *trachoma*, avascular superficial punctate keratitis (SPK) occurs.

In *herpes simplex* of secondary type (which usually occurs in adults), cornea is mostly involved. Minimal pain and lacrymation are met with. In this there are superficial spots in cornea (*SPK*) in rows which heal well, only to recur. In some cases, these may coalesce to form *dendritic* ulcer – a branched ulcer with knobs at the tip (Figs 6.d.4 and 6.d.5). Epithelium around the ulcer is loose and takes up *rose Bengal stain*. Dendritic ulcer may go onto amoeboid ulcer (*geographical ulcer*) in a few cases.

Treatment is by local use of IDU, Trifluridine (1%) drops or acyclovir (3%) ointment 5 times per day. If stroma is also involved

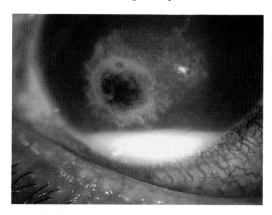

Figure 6.d.4: Dendritic ulcer due to herpes simplex virus

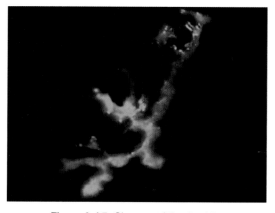

Figure 6.d.5: Close up of the dendrite

cortisone with antiviral drops are used. If epithelium is healthy and *only deeper layers of cornea* is affected then cortisone alone is used locally.

Herpes zoster is seen in adults. There is usually history of an attack of chicken pox in childhood. The virus is in Gasserian ganglion. If tip of nose is involved then eye is involved (*Hutchinson's rule*).

Herpes zoster ophthalmicus is mostly a unilateral condition. Severe pain over one side of face with redness followed by eruptions (vesicles) of skin is seen. It lasts for three weeks during which or after which eye signs appear. *Spots of* opacities in cornea and *dendritic* ulcer are the corneal lesions. Cornea is anaesthetic.

Management is with oral acyclovir (800/mg 5 times/day x 10 days) at the early stage of disease. Antibiotic ointment or calamine lotion is applied to skin lesions. Antibiotic ointment to eye is employed. Antiviral eye preparations locally are of no use. Local steroid is used for deep corneal lesions. Analgesics are must and sometimes even pethidine may be required.

Nursing

1. In herpes zoster the pain is sometimes so severe that the nurse must show a great concern and soothe the patient with encouraging words.
2. Cleanliness is important and infection to herself and to others must be avoided.
3. Skin condition must be dealt with properly.

EXPOSURE KERATITIS

It is *seen in* lagophthalmos (lids do not close properly) and the eye goes in for drying. Common *etiological factors* are seventh nerve paralysis, coma, very ill patients, marked symblepharon and severe proptosis (protrusion of eye ball). Such exposed cornea is affected by external noxious agents.

The condition starts as punctate spots just below the center of cornea which later on ulcerates due to invasion by organism.

Management is by keeping eyelids closed by suturing the lids together at the outer end (lateral tarsorrhaphy). If lagophthalmos is a temporary one, cornea is protected with antibiotic ointment.

Nursing

See under "Comatose patients" ("Nurse and ophthalmic patients")

INTERSTITIAL KERATITIS (IK)

It is an inflammation of corneal stroma *caused by* bacteria (especially of syphilis, Tuberculosis, leprosy), virus, fungus and protozoa. It is mostly an allergic reaction.

Syphilitic IK—It is met within congenital and occasionally in acquired syphilis. In congenital syphilis, the condition appears by 2nd decade of life and signs of congenital syphilis (including *Hutchinson's triad*) are seen. It is unilateral at a time, but finally affects both eyes. *Primary problem is iritis*. It starts as scattered infiltration (opacities) in corneal stroma at limbus and spreads to involve whole of cornea. Later vessels invade cornea in its deeper layers converting it into pinkish tissue. This clears up leaving behind vessels empty of blood and scattered opacities. Signs of iridocyclitis are seen. This is an allergic reaction to bacterial protein and not due to infection by bacteria.

Treatment is by local cycloplegic-mydriatic and steroids. Anti syphilitic treatment may be given; but has little influence on the local pathology or occurrence of the condition in the other eye later on. Local treatment should be continued for one year. If stopped earlier, recurrence occurs.

ARCUS SENILIS

It is a ring-shaped opacity near the limbus (corneo-scleral junction). There is a clear area between it and the limbus (Fig. 6.d.6). It is due to infiltration.

It starts by 6th decade of life. It starts at lower quadrant of cornea and later forms a ring. Blood cholesterol level has no bearing on it. If it occurs in young, it is known as arcus juvenilis.

Treatment is not needed for arcus senilis.

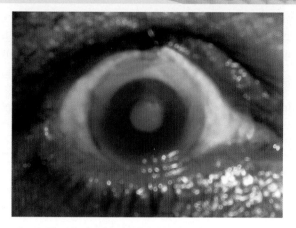

Figure 6.d.6: Arcus senilis

CORNEAL SCAR

It occurs after corneal injury, operations on cornea and corneal ulcer. Corneal opacity can also occur as a congenital phenomenon.

The opacity is of *three grades*:

1. *Nebula* – Least dense opacity. It can cause marked visual loss if centrally located.
2. *Macula*
3. *Leucoma* – Densest opacity (Figs 6.d.7 and 6.d.8).

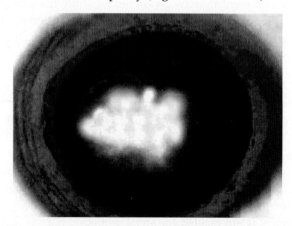

Figure 6.d.7: Leucoma. This is a corneal scar (Pupil is dilated)

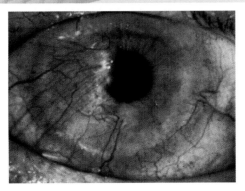

Figure 6.d.8: A corneal scar with plenty of vessels

Apart from cosmetic disfigurement, the main *symptom* of corneal scar is defective vision. This is either due to mechanical obstruction to rays of light (if the opacity is in the center of cornea), or due to change in the corneal curvature (if located peripherally). These opacities do not take up stain with 2% fluorescein. If iris is adherent to the opacity then the condition is called *adherent leucoma* (Fig. 6.d.9).

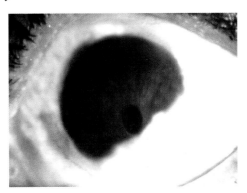

Figure 6.d.9: Adherent leucoma. The iris is adherent (attached) to the leucoma. The pupil is drawn down towards the leucoma

Management of corneal scar –
1. *Medical* therapy is useless.
2. Glasses or contact lens are useful for scars which are away from the center of cornea.
3. If the eye has no vision then tinted contact lens can be worn for cosmetic improvement.

4. Surgical:
   a. *Tattooing*—As scar is white in colour, it is easily seen by others. The aim of tattooing is to colour the scar so that its colour matches the color of iris behind.
   b. *Keratectomy*—In dense leucoma, the excess scar tissue is scraped off. Aim is to convert a leucoma into nebula. Visual improvement will not be much.
   c. *Optical iridectomy*—This is done for central scars. A small, keyhole-shaped opening is made in iris behind an area of clear cornea.
   d. *Keratoplasty*—The diseased portion of cornea (not the whole cornea) is removed and replaced with clear donor corneal piece (Figs 6.d.10 and 6.d.11).

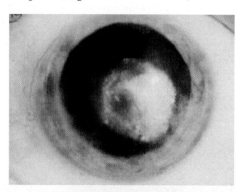

Figure 6.d.10: Leucoma

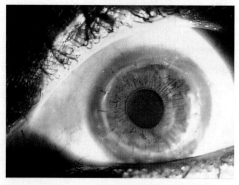

Figure 6.d.11: Case 6.d.10 for which a 8 mm penetrating corneal graft was done

CORNEAL GRAFTING (KERATOPLASTY)

This is popularly known as "eye transplantation". The donor material for keratoplasty is obtained within six hours of donor's death. Donor material is NEVER obtained from living persons. It is usually used within 24 hours. If preserved by special methods, the donor cornea can be used even after a week. Whole thickness of cornea (penetrating) or partial thickness of cornea (lamellar) is employed for grafting depending on the depth of corneal opacity. Whole cornea is not grafted. Usually not more than central 7 mm of cornea is replaced. It is done usually under local anaesthesia. Interrupted or continuous suture is employed (Fig. 6.d.12).

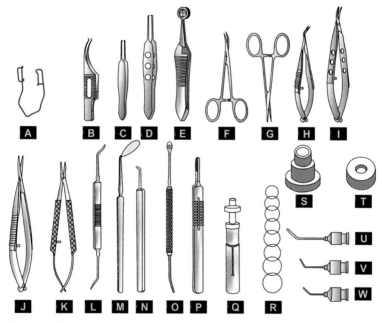

Figure 6.d.12: Instruments for keratoplasty. A – Barraquer wire speculum . B – Colibri forceps 1 X 2 Teeth. C – Bishop Harmon iris forceps. D – Mc Pherson corneal forceps 1 X 2 Teeth. E – Dastoor corneal graft holding Forceps. F – Hartman mosquito forceps (Curved). G – Hartman mosquito forceps (Stright). H – Vannas capsulotomy scissors angled. I – Corneal scissors universal. J – Westcott tenotomy scissors. K – Barraquer needle holder (Micro). L – Castroviejo cyclodialysis spatula. M – Dastoor keratoplasty spatula. N – Paufique graft knife. O – Paton spatula and spoon. P – B.P. handle. Q – Castroviejo corneal trephine. R – Flieringa scleral fixation Rings. S – Tudor Thomas corneal graft stand. T – Lieberman teflon block. U – Viscoelastic cannula. V – Bishop Harmon A/C cannula. W – Air injection cannula (27G).

Apart from optical purpose, corneal grafting is *done* for therapeutic, cosmetic and tectonic (to restore the thickness of cornea) purposes also. Best results are obtained with avascular central leucoma, keratoconus and corneal dystrophy.

Cortisone is given postoperatively for a month. Graft rejection due to immune reaction is the common problem. Other complications are – vessels invading the graft, infection, glaucoma, graft edema, iritis and anterior synechia (attachment of iris) to wound.

Nursing

1. Nurse should have a thorough knowledge about corneal grafting.
2. She must dispel the wrong idea in the minds of the patient that the whole eyeball can be replaced and that it is useful even in eye with no light perception or dead, shrunken eye.
3. Some parents might approach to donate their own eyes for their child while they themselves are alive. She must tell that, unlike kidney donation, eyes are removed only after a person dies and that too within 6 hours.
4. The successful outcome depends upon so many factors including the type of corneal disease, size of lesion, vessels in cornea, the condition of iris and anterior chamber.
5. Postoperatively, patient must have local drops regularly.
6. Nurse must advise the patient not to strain for at least a month.
7. She must warn the patient that any direct injury to the eye may result in the rupture of the graft wound even after years.

KERATOCONUS

It is otherwise known as conical cornea. It is mostly a congenital condition which manifests by second decade of life. In this condition, the cornea slowly protrudes like a cone (Fig. 6.d.13). It produces defective vision.

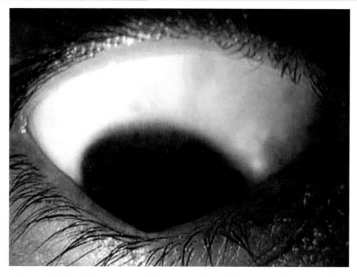

Figure 6.d.13: Keratoconus. When the patient looks down, the protruding cornea makes a 'dent' in the lower lid (as in this photo).

The cone is near the center of cornea. Early diagnosis is by Placido disc, keratometry, distant direct ophthalmoscope and by corneal topography. In a few cases the cornea turns opaque due to inflow of aqueous into cornea caused by Descemet's membrane rupture.

Management is with glasses or contact lens in early stage and by keratoplasty (usually penetrating) in later stages. Result of corneal grafting is very good.

INJURIES

Mechanical injury to cornea is an emergency. The eye should be immediately patched with antibiotics, ophthalmologist informed and tests needed for general anaesthesia done. Patient should be asked not to take anything by mouth. X-ray may be needed.

In lime burns, the nurse must *Immediately* wash the eye with at least one pint of saline (or any water). Local anaesthetic drops may be used. She should not wait for the doctor (Fig. 6.d.14).

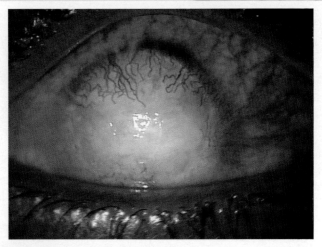

Figure 6.d.14: Case of lime burns. This case has a very poor prognosis.

(e) SCLERA

Scleritis, episcleritis (inflammation of sclera and episcleral tissue) and staphyloma are common scleral conditions.

Sclera can be studied through conjunctiva only. Swelling, thinning and discolouration are to be noted down.

EPISCLERITIS

It is mostly an allergic manifestation to endogenous toxin. It is seen with collagen diseases.

Young adults, mostly females, are affected. Pain may or may not be present. Usually it occurs temporal to cornea and has an acute onset. It is seen as red patch in one or both eyes with mild tenderness (Fig. 6.e.1). It may be either diffuse or nodular lesion. It recurs. Except for its recurrence and chronicity, the only other problem is the slate colour scar to which conjunctiva is adherent.

Treatment is difficult.
1. Mild to strong steroids are used locally.

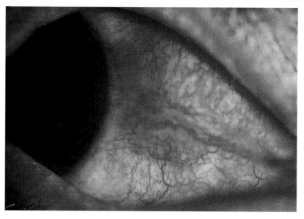

Figure 6.e.1: Episcleritis

2. Oral NSAID is useful. NSAID is also used locally instead of steroids. This can avoid problems of long-term use of local steroids (Glaucoma, cataract and secondary infection). Oral salicylate and ibuprofen are sometimes used.
3. Cold compress applied locally gives relief from symptoms.

SCLERITIS

It is like episcleritis; but involves deeper tissue. It is a bilateral, chronic condition. It is seen with connective tissue, collagen disorders, metabolic disorders like gout, syphilis, infection by bacteria such as *staphylococcus*, ocular surgery and herpes zoster.

It is present either in the anterior or posterior region. *Anterior scleritis*, which is associated with above disorders, can manifest as nodular, diffuse or necrotising *type*. Necrotising scleritis with inflammation presents as red, painful eye with severe symptoms. Scleral thinning, glaucoma, cataract and corneal melt are seen.

Diffuse scleritis is pink in colour. In contrast, *nodular scleritis* is an elevated purple nodule at limbus (corneo-scleral junction).

Posterior scleritis is a local manifestation only and produces decreased vision, reduced ocular movements and proptosis. Pain may or may not be present. B scan and CT scan assist in its diagnosis.

Management begins with thorough investigations.

Treatment

1. It is mainly systemic – NSAID, steroids and, if needed, immunosuppressants. Ranitidine is given along with this therapy.
2. If infective element is present, local and systemic antibiotics are warranted.
3. If scleral perforation occurs, scleral patch graft is done.

STAPHYLOMA

Staphyloma is protrusion of cornea or sclera lined by uveal tissue. Except for anterior type, the other types involve sclera in which *scleral thinning* is a must. The thinning may be due to scleral inflammation, degeneration, surgery, trauma or stretching of eye globe.

The various *types* of staphyloma are:

a. *Anterior staphyloma*—It is seen after a slow perforation of a large corneal ulcer. The uveal tissue involved is iris.
b. *Intercalary staphyloma*—It is seen within 2 mm of limbus (corneoscleral junction). The protruding portion of sclera is lined by root of iris and anterior part of ciliary body.
c. *Ciliary staphyloma*—It is seen from 2 mm to 8 mm from limbus. The tissue lining is ciliary body (Fig. 6.e.2).

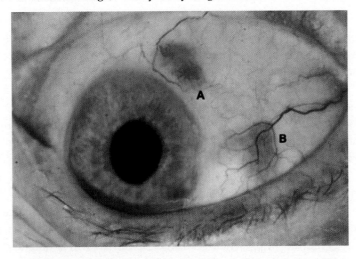

Figure 6.e.2: Staphyloma. Intercalary (A) and ciliary staphyloma (B)

d. *Equatorial staphyloma*—This occurs 14 mm behind limbus. It is lined by choroid and is seen in high myopia also.

e. *Posterior staphyloma*—It is seen in high myopia, after scleritis and injuries. The sclera is lined by choroid. The diagnosis is by funduscopy.

Management

1. *Prevention* and treatment of factors causing scleral thinning need attention.
2. Once it has occurred, local *excision and repair* with scleral graft are done.
3. Posterior staphyloma may require *scleral support* procedure. If high myopia is present, glasses are prescribed.

(f) UVEAL TRACT

Iridocyclitis is an important clinical condition.

Proper examination of iris requires oblique illumination and slit-lamp study. Retro illumination is sometimes employed. Gonioscopy (to see angle of A/C) study is done to examine the extreme periphery of iris.

Pupil is examined for direct and indirect (consensual) reactions, size and shape.

The common pathology of uveal tract is inflammation. They are also affected by new growth.

INFLAMMATION (UVEITIS)

Uveitis is divided into anterior (which involves iris and ciliary body) and posterior (in which choroid is involved). Anterior Uveitis is known as Iridocyclitis.

Panophthalmitis is an acute purulent inflammation of whole uveal tract caused by purulent organisms which gain entrance from outside or from surrounding tissues. Patient has severe pain, proptosis (protrusion of eyeball) and total loss of vision. Cornea sloughs off and the whole eyeball is filled with pus.

Management is by removal of eyeball (evisceration), higher antibiotics and analgesics.

IRIDOCYCLITIS

It is a common condition of uveal tract. The cause might be allergy to airborne allergen or to microbial antigen of TB, streptococcus.

Infection is another cause. Bacteria, parasite, virus or fungus may be the cause. They may invade either from outside or from contiguous structure such as cornea and sclera, or from an endogenous focus.

Some of the cases are caused by *toxins* which may be bacterial, autotoxin, from ocular tissue or chemical substance.

HLA B27 *antigen* is frequently associated with this condition.

Rarely ocular *trauma* can cause this.

It is grouped into granulomatous and nongranulomatous types.

Affecting any age group and any gender, the intensity of symptoms varies between granulomatous and nongranulomatous types. The signs also depend upon the reaction that the inflammation produces – cellular, serous or purulent.

Symptoms include defective vision, pain in the eye, Headache and glaring.

The signs are: Cells in anterior chamber and vitreous. The iris shows change in colour and loss of its pattern (Fig. 6.f.1). It may get stuck to

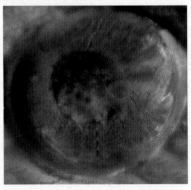

Figure 6.f.1: Thin exudate over the pupil in a case of iritis

the lens partially or totally (Fig. 6.f.2). In many cases, the lens shows cataract. The intraocular pressure may go up. In severe cases, the intraocular pressure drops and the eye may get shrunken.

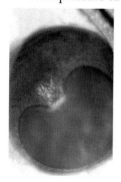

Figure 6.f.2: Case with posterior synechia (Sticking of one point of pupil border to lens). (Local pupillary dilating drug has been applied).

The condition may spread behind to the choroid resulting in choroiditis. In some cases the optic nerve also can get involved.

Acute iridocyclitis has to be differentiated from acute conjunctivitis and acute angle closure glaucoma (Table 6.f.1).

Table 6.f.1: Main differential diagnosis of iridocyclitis			
	Acute conjunctivitis	*Acute iridocyclitis*	*Acute congestive glaucoma*
1. Cause	Infection	Allergy, infection	Angle closure
2. Onset	Sudden	Sudden	Sudden
3. Pain	+	++	+++
4. Congestion	Conjunctival	Ciliary	Ciliary
5. Vision	Normal	Reduced	Markedly reduced
6. Discharge	++	+ (watery)	+ (watery)
7. Halos	+	–	+
8. Tenderness	–	++	++
9. Cornea	Clear	Clear or hazy	Hazy
10. A/C	Normal	Variable	Very shallow depth
11. Iris	Normal	Minimal haziness +	No change
12. Pupil	Normal	Small, sluggish	Dilated; sluggish
13. Media	Clear	Hazy	Hazy
14. IOP	Normal	Variable	Very much raised

Perhaps a word about "red eye" is appropriate at this point:

Table 6.f.2: Differential diagnosis of the red eye

	Acute Conjunctivitis	Acute Iritis	Acute Glaucoma	Corneal ulcer or Trauma	Scleritis	Episcleritis
Dilated Vessels	Near fornix	Around cornea	Around cornea	Around cornea	Local	Local
Pupil	Not affected	Small	Large	Small or normal	Normal	Normal
Increased IOP	—	May be seen	Marked	—	—	—
Opacity of cornea	—	Cornea hazy	Cornea hazy	Steamy Cornea Opacity +	—	—
Ocular Discharge	Purulent	Watery	Watery	Purulent	—	—
Decreased Vision	—	Yes	Yes	Yes	—	—
Pain	+	++	+++	++	+	+
Prognosis	Self Limited; 3-5 Days	MAY BE EXTEREMELY SERIOUS WITHOUT PROPER TREATMENT				Self Limited 2 – 4 Weeks

MANAGEMENT

Investigations for syphilis, TB, leprosy and arthritis, HLA – B27, ANA, PTA – ABS, ACE, RPR and X-ray should be carried out.

I. Treatment for the *causative* disease.
II. Specific treatment:
   1. Pupillary *dilatation* with drops, ointment or injection of atropine under the conjunctiva.
   2. *Locally corticosteroid*–Beta–methasone or prednisolone as drops, ointment or via subtenon route is used.
   3. In cases where topical route is ineffective or in very severe cases, *systemic steriod* or *periocular* methylprednisolone is used.
   4. If there is no response with this therapy, *systemic immunosuppressant* such as methotrexate is given.
   5. *Local* warm application and oral aspirin to relieve the *pain*. Former increases local circulation.
   6. Dark glasses.

Nursing

1. The Nurse must emphasise to the patient the importance of the various investigations that are to be carried out.

2. She must encourage the patient with soothing words. In spite of treatment some cases go in for blindness slowly.
3. She must tell the patient the various problems with long term use of local cortisone (local as well as systemic).
4. Since the treatment is prolonged in a few cases, she must see to it that the patient uses the medicines regularly.

SYMPATHETIC OPHTHALMIA (SO)

It is a granulomatous iridocyclitis of both eyes with immune etiology. The antigen is uveal pigment. It is a bilateral condition in which the normal (sympathising) eye suffers from uveitis when the other (exciting) eye is injured. This is seen if the exciting eye is injured over ciliary body area which is known as the *danger zone of eye* (area between 2 and 4 mm from limbus), or rarely after an intraocular surgery. It is common if uveal tissue is incarcerated in the wound.

In both the eyes, the uveal tract is heavily infiltrated by lymphocytes and plasma cells. There is proliferation of pigment epithelium (of iris and ciliary body) forming Dalen-Fuchs nodules. Caseation is absent.

The *CLINICAL PICTURE* is characterised by the non-subsidence of iridocyclitis in the exciting eye. There is retention of some vision in it. The *onset* is usually two weeks after injury. If the injured eye is shrunken and blind, irritation returns in it with the onset of SO. In the other (sympathising) eye, photophobia and difficulty in near vision are the earliest *symptoms.* Tenderness is present in both eyes. The full blown picture is that of bilateral (granulomatous) iridocyclitis.

In the *MANAGEMENT*, *prevention* is the best. The penetrating wound must be properly treated–incarcerated tissue released and wound properly sutured. Antibiotics and cortisone are given. If the injured eye is to be removed it should be done *within a fortnight*.

Once the *disease has set in*, if the exciting eye has no vision, it should be removed in the early stage. If the exciting eye has some vision it should be retained since, after the disease subsides, the injured (exciting) eye may sometimes retain useful vision while sympathising eye will have none. The treatment is local pupillary dilators and systemic steroid – intravenous to begin with. If steroids cannot be given or ineffective, oral Cyclosporine A is useful. This drug can also be given along with steroids. It should be remembered that local steroid *must be used for about 18 months* – the normal duration of the disease. If stopped early, SO recurs.

SIDEROSIS BULBI

It is a post traumatic condition in which an iron alloy (iron less than 85%) is retained inside the eye. In this condition, the iris color changes to green and then reddish brown. Lens shows a rusty ring and cataract changes.

Management—It is early removal of the foreign body.

Copper alloy produces *chalcosis* in which sunflower cataract and Kayser—Fleischer ring of cornea are seen.

IRIDECTOMY

This is the process by which a piece of iris is removed either surgically or by laser. The various types of iridectomy and their indications are (Fig. 6.f.3): a) *Peripheral iridectomy*–Along with corneal grafting,

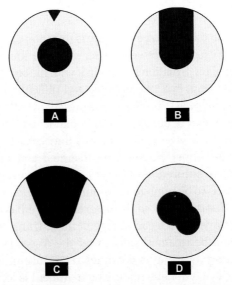

Figure 6.f.3: Types of Iridectomy. A – Peripheral iridectomy. B – Complete (sector) iridectomy. C – Broad basal iridectomy. D – Optical iridectomy.

cataract and glaucoma surgeries and in first three stages of narrow angle glaucoma. b) *Complete (sector) iridectomy*–Along with cataract surgery, for extensive posterior synechiae, retinal detachment in the other eye, possible long-term miotic therapy, sphincter rigidity and in iridencleisis, c) *Broad basal iridectomy*–Prophylaxis for hemorrhagic glaucoma. d) *Optical (key hole) iridectomy*–Central leucoma and central, stationary, congenital cataract, e) *Iris excision*–Impacted foreign body in iris (especially chemically active one), infected iris prolapse and tumors of iris (amount of iris excised depends upon the size of the pathology).

NEOVASCULARISATION OF IRIS

In this condition, new vessels grow over the iris which can be seen with slit lamp. This is met with in iritis and retinal condition such as diabetic retinopathy, central retinal vein occlusion.

These new vessels may grow across the angle and block the exit of aqueous. This leads to rise in ocular pressure (secondary glaucoma). Sometimes bleeding occurs into anterior chamber (Hyphema) which again can cause glaucoma.

IRIDODIALYSIS

It is the separation of iris from its root. It is usually *due to* trauma – either injury or operative.

The patient may rarely *complain* of diplopia. He may also have (in blue iris) cosmetic complaint. Glaring is a rare symptom.

Examination shows that the pupil is D shaped. The dialysed portion of the pupil is seen near the limbus and it appears dark (Fig. 6.f.4).

Treatment is usually not required. If symptom is marked, the detached portion of the iris periphery can be anchored to the root with 10/0 suture.

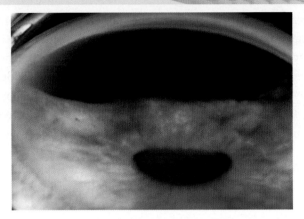

Figure 6.f.4: Iridodialysis. The area where iris is detached from its root is seen in superior aspect. Pupil is D-shaped

(g) LENS

Diseases of lens are most common. Hence it is important that the nurse has thorough knowledge of the diseases of lens as well as the treatment procedures.

Lens is examined with diffuse illumination, oblique illumination and slit lamp. Opacities of lens, if present, must be carefully studied for its morphology.

CATARACT

Cataract is the opacity of the cortex, nucleus and sometimes capsule of the lens. It is classified into developmental and acquired–the latter into senile and complicated. Usually developmental cataract is mostly partial and stationary; while acquired is progressive.

1. SENILE (AGE RELATED) CATARACT

The **etiology** is still obscure. Hereditary, doing near work for a long time, sunlight and UV radiation are implicated.

In senile cataract, there are two *varieties*–cortical and nuclear, depending upon where the opacity starts to develop. In *nuclear cataract,* sclerosis of nucleus is the main change. Deposition of pigments may give it a dark brown or even black colour. But, *cortical cataract* formation goes through many *stages*. To begin with fluid gets into lens. In some cases the hydration causes swelling of lens (*intumescent stage cataract*) resulting in shallowing of anterior chamber. If the patient has pre existing shallow anterior chamber then sometimes raised ocular pressure occurs. This requires immediate surgery.

In the next stage (*incipient stage*) wedge shaped opacities are seen in lens periphery. They are in cortex situated behind as well as in front of nucleus.

The next two stages are *immature and mature cataract stages*. Their differentiation is given below (Table 6.g.1):

Table 6.g.1: Differences between immature and mature cataracts		
	Immature	*Mature*
Clear lens fibers	Seen in some areas	No clear lens fibers
Iris shadow	Present	Absent
Color (Cortical)	Grey	Pearly White
Vision	Some Vision +	Only PL +
Ophthalmoscopy	Black shadow in red reflex	Only black shadow

(The above differences are for senile cortical cataract only).

The cause of iris shadow is the presence of a few clear lens fibers between the capsule of lens and the cataractous area.

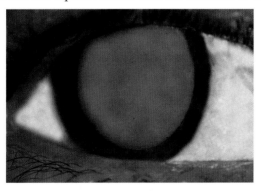

Figure 6.g.1: Mature cataract (Pupil is dilated)

The final stage is *hypermature* one. In this stage the hypermature cataract presents in various ways.

a. *Morgagnian cataract*–The cortex liquefies into a white fluid in which the brown nucleus sinks down. In some cases it can lead to uveitis and glaucoma due to lens cortical matter that has leaked out (Fig. 6.g.2).

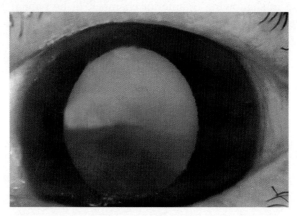

Figure 6.g.2: Morgagnian hypermature cataract. The cortex is liquefied (white area) and the nucleus has sunk down (brown area)

b. The whole lens may shrink causing iridodonesis and some amount of deepening of anterior chamber.
c. The lens may be subluxated or dislocated due to degeneration of zonule fibers. It may result in secondary glaucoma.

The prominent *symptom* is

1. *Defective distant vision* which is more marked during day time in nuclear cataract. In cortical cataract the defect is more during the night time. Later on, distance vision deteriorates with growth of cataract, finally ending in light perception only.

The other symptoms are

2. *Near vision* improves in some cases. The patient might be able to read without the aid of near vision glasses which he had been using. This is called "second vision" or "second sight"
3. Some patients complain of black, fixed *spots* in the field of vision.
4. Coloured *haloes* are seen by a few.
5. Some experience a minimal *red tinge* in their vision.
6. Glare by light is the most discomforting symptom.
7. Frequent change of glasses.

Management is mainly surgical.
1. Any *medical treatment* will not dissolve lens opacity.
2. Spectacles are useful in early stages. Mydriatic may be used. In modern days, surgery is done even at (early) immature stage.
3. *Surgery* can either be intracapsular (ICCE) (whole lens with capsule removed) (Fig. 6.g.3) or extracapsular (ECCE) (Posterior capsule of lens is left behind in eye and rest of lens portion–cortex and nucleus–removed) extraction.

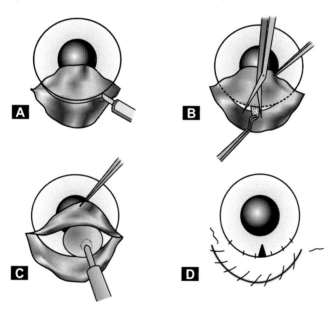

Figure 6.g.3: Steps of ICCE. A – Limbal incision (opening) made. B – Iridectomy performed. C – Lens removed in toto with cryo equipment. D – Limbal and conjunctival wounds closed

Before surgery is taken up, projection of light should be checked. General state of patient must be assessed especially for hypertension and diabetes. Local and systemic focus of infection must be looked for and eliminated.

Preoperatively, pupil is dilated, intraocular pressure lowered with acetazolamide, ocular massage done, and minimal sedation given.

The operation is done either under general or local anaesthesia. In the latter technique, facial and retrobulbar blocks are used.

Peribulbar is another method that is employed. This method does not require facial block.

In ECCE, the lens cortical material and the nucleus are removed after opening the anterior capsule. Iridectomy usually is not done (Fig. 6.g.4). There are so many variations in surgery. ECCE is popular nowadays since it facilitates placing *intraocular lens* (IOL) at the end of surgery.

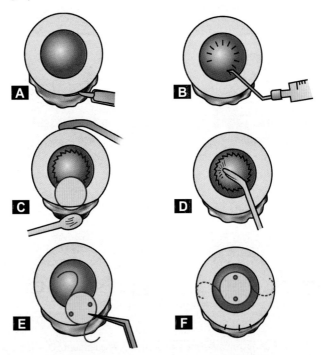

Figure 6.g.4: ECCE steps. A – Limbal opening made. B – Anterior lens capsule incisions ("can opener" method) made. C – The nucleus expressed out through the anterior capsule and limbal openings. D – The cortical matter aspirated. E – The IOL is introduced into A/C. F – The IOL haptics are placed in the horizontal position and limbal wound closed

IOL (intraocular lens) is made of PMMA, acrylic or silicone. It has a central disc called optic and two limbs called haptics. IOL may have holes in the optics (called dialing hole) or may not have the holes (Fig. 6.g.5). The IOL may be placed at three places inside the eye: a) Behind iris (posterior chamber lens; P/C IOL), b) Attached to iris (iris clip on lens) (Fig. 6.g.6), or c) in anterior chamber in front of iris (anterior chamber lens; A/C IOL) (Figs 6.g.7 and 6.g.8). A/C IOL is employed after ICCE or if IOL is inserted at a latter date after cataract surgery. Generally A/C IOL is not much preferred because of the possibility of damage to cornea and loss of vision. For P/C IOL to remain in position inside the eye, it should be supported by posterior capsule of lens behind (which is possible only with ECCE). Otherwise IOL will slip into vitreous.

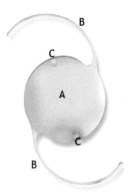

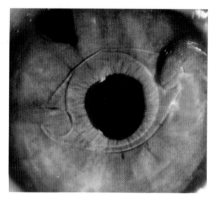

Figure 6.g.5: Posterior Chamber IOL (P/C IOL). IOL is placed behind the iris. It has a round central optic (A) and two supporting arms haptics; (B). Some models have dialing holes (C)

Figure 6.g.6: IOL attached to iris (Iris-clip-on lens)

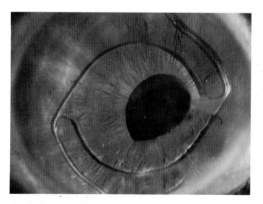

Figure 6.g.7: Anterior chamber IOL (A/C IOL). It can cause damage to cornea and loss of vision

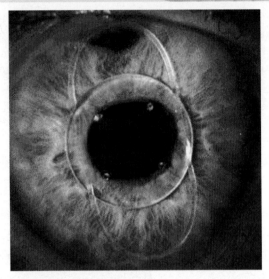

Figure 6.g.8: Another model of A/C IOL

The power of P/C IOL is around + 19. But the exact power that is needed is calculated (using SRK formula) after measuring the length of eyeball with A-scan (Fig. 6.g.9).

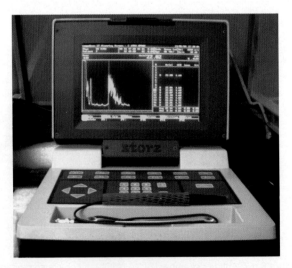

Figure 6.g.9: A-scan which is used to measure the length of eyeball

An eye from which lens has been removed and IOL is placed is known as *pseudophakia*.

Complications

1. Posterior capsule opacification (*PCO*) is a common postoperative problem after ECCE. Opening is made in the opaque capsule by Nd: YAG laser capsulotomy.
2. *Hyphema* (Blood in anterior chamber)–It usually gets absorbed. Rarely it may require evacuation if it persists beyond seven days.
3. *Infection*–Prevention is the best.
4. *Retinal detachment*–It is common with ICCE.

The recent surgical techniques for cataract are Small Incision Cataract Surgery (SICS) and phacoemulsification.

2. DEVELOPMENTAL CATARACT

It occurs at birth or later. The *etiology* is not definitely known in all cases. a) Virus, especially rubella, b) deficient oxygenation to fetus due to placental hemorrhage, c) maternal malnutrition involving vitamin D, d) radiation e) hypocalcemia and f) infant malnutrition are some of the causes. g) In some cases, hereditary factor plays a role.

Most of developmental cataracts do not attract the attention of patients as they do not cause defective vision due to their peripheral location. So patients with this peripheral type of congenital cataracts may not have any visual problem and do not need treatment.

Symptoms are mostly present with centrally located ones. They cause defective vision, white opacity in pupillary area (leucocoria), nystagmus and squint. Opacity may involve anterior capsule, anterior cortex, nucleus, posterior cortex, posterior capsule and even whole lens. It occurs as punctate cataract (blue dot, sutural cataract or dots in the nucleus), coronary cataract (in the periphery as club shaped opacities), coralliform cataract, anterior cortical, anterior pyramidal cataract, disc-shaped opacity in posterior cortex or as total cataract. The more important variety is zonular cataract.

Zonular (Lamellar) cataract is the commonest (50%) of all developmental cataracts. It can either be due to hereditary (dominant) factor or to malnutrition, especially vitamin D. The fibers that develop during period of malnutrition are opaque, while fibers that develop before and after this period are clear and transparent. So, the opaque fibers are buried in the middle of clear lens areas. The opacity is seen as a disc-shaped one (from in front) with riders going out (Fig. 6.g.10). Associated transverse lines on permanent incisors and canine teeth are present.

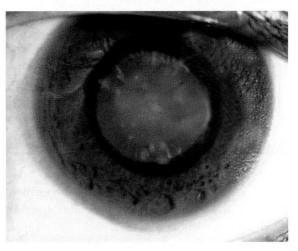

Figure 6.g.10: Lamellar cataract (Zonular cataract). This is a developmental cataract seen in children due to vitamin D deficiency in mother during pregnancy

In the *management* of congenital cataract, preliminary detailed examination and investigations are important.

Treatment is carried out only if vision is grossly affected. If possible, in central cataract with clear periphery, the surgery should be postponed till puberty.

In lamellar cataract, operation should be deferred till the child is at least two years old; Till then pupil can be kept dilated with local use of mydriatic. Earlier surgery is done if pupil does not dilate or if lens opacity involves the whole lens and if there is nystagmus or squint.

The *techniques* used are–a) Lensectomy (No PCO, but retinal detachment may occur), b) lens aspiration with anterior vitrectomy (Less PCO; for children below two years) and c) simple lens aspiration (best for IOL implantation).

3. ACQUIRED CATARACT

It can be *due to* diseases of eye, systemic condition or to injury. Most of these cataracts have polychromatic (multicolour appearance) lusture. Vision is affected early.

Diseases of anterior segment of eye such as corneal ulcer and iridocyclitis and those due to *posterior segment* lesions such as choroiditis, retinal detachment, retinitis pigmentosa can produce such a cataract. The *systemic diseases* associated with acquired cataract are diabetes, hypoparathyroid and certain skin diseases.

In *diabetics*, the cataract develops earlier and faster and has *"snowflake like"* appearance.

Trauma–Mechanical (Fig. 6.g.11), chemical and radiational and toxic substances such as dinitrophenol, thalium, strong miotics, steroids and cyanate can result in cataract formation.

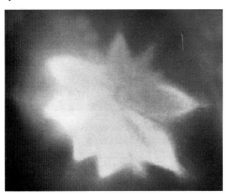

Figure 6.g.11: Traumatic cataract

Cataract due to infrared (heat) is seen in glass workers. Radiation and powerful electric current also cause cataract.

Treatment, except that for the causative factor, is essentially similar to senile cataract.

AFTER CATARACT (SECONDARY CATARACT)

This type of cataract is usually met with after ECCE. Immediately after surgery the patient has good vision; then it starts going down slowly. The *various types (causes)* are:

1. The commonest type is *posterior capsular opacification (PCO)* in which the transparent posterior capsule that is left behind after ECCE slowly becomes opaque. Vision is impaired.
2. Formation of ring-like "cataract" behind the iris—*Ring of Sommering*. Vision is not impaired.
3. In certain situation, the remnant epithelial cells under anterior capsule form balloon-like cells instead of lens fibers. These occupy the pupillary area and appear like pearls (*Elschnig's pearls*) (Fig. 6.g.12). Vision may be impaired.

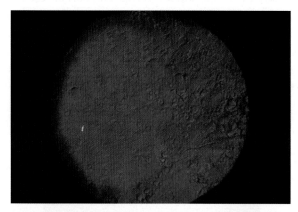

Figure 6.g.12: Elschnig's pearls. This is one type of after (secondary) cataract which is met with following extracapsular cataract extraction surgery.

Management is by making an opening in the *after cataract* by instrumental needling (using Ziegler knife), by vitreous cutter or by Nd: YAG laser. This is needed only if the vision is affected.

SUBLUXATION AND DISLOCATION OF LENS (ECTOPIA LENTIS)

A lens is said to be subluxated or dislocated if it is not in its usual anatomical position either completely or partially. The lens may be in anterior chamber, caught in the pupil or in vitreous (Fig. 6.g.13).

The *causes* are: 1) Congenital, 2) traumatic, 3) ocular conditions, 4) certain systemic conditions (Marfan's, Weil-Marchesani and homocystinuria) and 5. Couching.

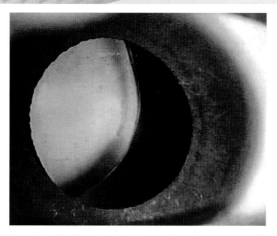

Figure 6.g.13: Posteriorly subluxated lens. It can cause rise in intraocular pressure, iritis and retinal detachment

Ocular conditions that can cause subluxation are high myopia, buphthalmos (a type of congenital glaucoma), keratoglobus (big cornea), aniridia, Reiger's anomaly, uveitis and degenerative status inside the eye including hypermaturity of cataract.

Couching is the method used by itinerant mendicants to treat cataract by depressing the lens with a needle passed into eye through limbus or sclera. It is not seen nowaday due to government steps to eradicate cataract.

Anterior subluxation results in secondary glaucoma.

Symptoms: In subluxation, there may not be any symptoms. Or, defective vision, glare and uniocular polyopia (multiple vision) may occur.

Management of anterior dislocation and pupil incarcerated lens is surgical removal of it. The same is for posterior dislocation if there is complication. Otherwise spectacles are given for posterior dislocation. The aphakic area is corrected.

APHAKIA

It is absence of lens from its normal position, i.e. pupillary area. The *cause* can be a) congenital (Very rare cause), or due to b) trauma and c) surgery. Patient has defective vision for both distance and near.

The *signs* are deep anterior chamber, iridodonesis (tremulousness of iris due to loss of normal support by iris) and jet black pupil. Evidence of operation, iridectomy and after cataract may be seen (Fig. 6.g.14). In pseudophakia, IOL is seen. The anterior chamber is normal in pseudophakic eye with posterior chamber IOL.

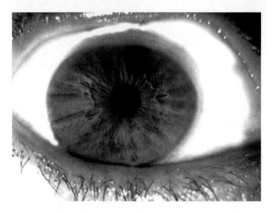

Figure 6.g.14: Aphakia with peripheral iridectomy. The pupillary area is dark. There is no IOL in this case

Treatment is to substitute the missing lens by spectacles, contact lens, IOL or refractive surgery (if the power is low). Now aphakic spectacle has been almost totally replaced by IOL. Even with latter, near vision needs spectacle correction. But multifocal IOL has obliterated the use of spectacle completely. Table 6.g.1 compares these treatment modalities.

Table 6.g.1: Comparison of certain Aphakic correction			
	Aphakic Correction with		
	Spectacle	*Contact lens*	*IOL*
Discomfort	++	+ (of cleaning)	Nil
Increase in image	35%	8%	1%
Diplopia (if other eye is normal)	+	No	No
Fields	Restricted	Normal	Normal
Cosmetic disfigurement	+	No	No
Handling by patient	Easy	Difficult	Not required

INJURIES

Injuries to lens are for the ophthalmologist to deal with. In fact he is in a better position to diagnose that the lens is damaged. One important fact that a nurse should remember is that, sometimes, the lens damage after injury may manifest itself after some days or even weeks.

(h) GLAUCOMA

Glaucoma is increase in intraocular pressure resulting in damage to optic nerve and finally loss of sight. Examination for a case of glaucoma requires many instruments – Anterior segment should be examined with slit lamp and intraocular pressure (IOP) is measured with tonometer–either with Schiotz or Goldmann applanation tonometer. Corneal thickness is assessed with pachymeter and the angle of anterior chamber with gonioscope. Fundus study is by direct and indirect ophthalmoscope with or without fluorescein angiography. Field study is by static perimetry (Fig. 6.h.1).

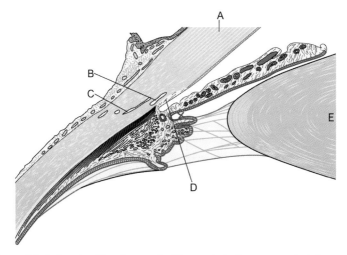

Figure 6.h.1: Anterior Chamber angle. The angle is the outer end of the space between iris and cornea (marked with X in the photo). A – Cornea. B – Schlemm's canal. C – Drainage channel. D – Trabecular meshwork (TMW). Through this angle and trabecular meshwork the aqueous goes out of the eye. E – Lens

Knowledge of anatomy of angle of anterior chamber is a must to understand glaucoma.

Etiology

The cause of glaucoma is a) obstruction to the outflow of aqueous (at pupil, anterior chamber (A/C) angle or aqueous vein) or b) excess secretion of aqueous. Such an increase in ocular pressure presses on the whole of eyeball coat; but the weakest point gives way – this point being optic disc. The disc and the nerve fibers of retina are damaged. The optic disc damage can also occur even with normal intraocular pressure (IOP).

Normal intraocular pressure is 10 mm/Hg to 21mm/Hg. This is measured by Schiotz tonometer (which can give false reading if there is change in scleral rigidity) (Figs 6.h.2 and 6.h.3) or with applanation tonometer (which gives more accurate reading) (Fig. 6.h.4).

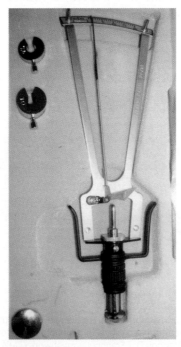

Figure 6.h.2: Schiotz tonometer. Popular one; but may give false value of intraocular pressure (IOP) in a few cases

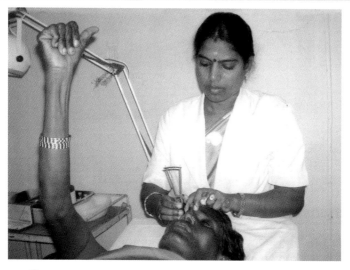

Figure 6.h.3: Tonometry (measuring IOP) with Schiotz tonometer

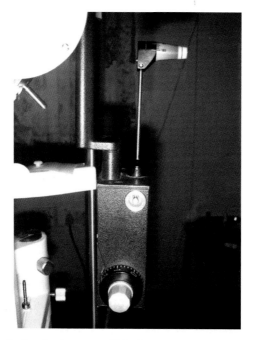

Figure 6.h.4: Applanation tonometer. This gives accurate measurement of IOP

There are many *classifications* of glaucoma. The simplest one is:

1. Congenital

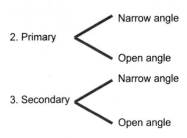

2. Primary — Narrow angle
— Open angle

3. Secondary — Narrow angle
— Open angle

"CONGENITAL" GLAUCOMA

This usually means primary congenital glaucoma which is otherwise known as buphthalmos or hydrophthalmia.

Primary Congenital Glaucoma

It is *due to* failure of iris to separate completely from cornea so that A/C is not communicating with trabecular meshwork. It is a hereditary disease. Male: Female = 3:2. Glaucoma occurs within two years of life. It is a bilateral (75%) condition. The parents notice that the eye is larger, that cornea is hazy (Fig. 6.h.5), and that the child has glaring and watering from eye.

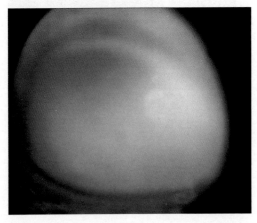

Figure 6.h.5: Cornea of a case of congenital glaucoma

Examination shows increase in corneal diameter and curvature, deep A/C, and thinning of sclera near limbus. The eye is myopic. Fundus shows increase in optic disc cup. At the end stage vision is totally lost.

Treatment is surgical only. Goniotomy, trabeculotomy or, if these two fail, trabeculectomy is recommended.

PRIMARY GLAUCOMAS

They are called primary because they are not secondary to any other ocular, systemic or traumatic causes. They are of two *types*– narrow and open angle.

Narrow (Closed) Angle Glaucoma

In this condition, the A/C is shallow and its angle is less than 20° i.e. narrow (Fig. 6.h.6). When the patient reaches the 5th decade of life or so, the shallowness worsens due to increase in thickness of lens (Fig. 6.h.7). In such a situation, if pupil dilates due to any cause, the iris gets bunched up at the angle. The angle gets closed totally, aqueous flow gets blocked (Fig. 6.h.8). Intra ocular pressure (IOP) goes up. It is more common in females and in adults in 5th decade of life and after.

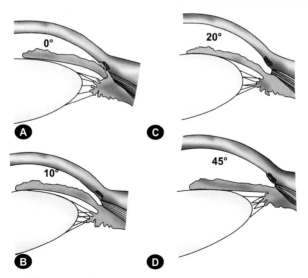

Figure 6.h.6: Comparison of angle of A/C in narrow angle (A) and open angle (D) eyes

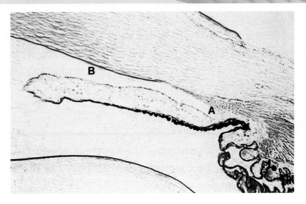

Figure 6.h.7: Specimen of a case of narrow angle glaucoma.
A – Angle. B – Anterior chamber

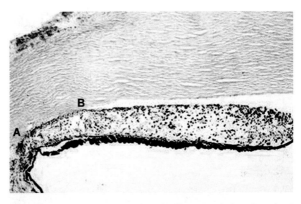

Figure 6.h.8: Pathological specimen (slide) of a case of closed angle glaucoma.
Angle and anterior chamber are closed from A to B

In the evolution of narrow angle glaucoma there are five *stages.*
In the first two stages persons have discomfort now and then with
coloured haloes and blurring of vision. These later on occur
constantly. If pupil is dilated in these cases (such as application of
pupil dilating drops) *Acute congestive glaucoma* occurs. It is seen more
in ladies above the age of 40. It is usually unilateral at a time; but
simultaneous bilateral occurrence is also met with. It is due to the
iris bunching up at the angle and obstructing the out flow of aqueous.
The IOP goes up. Systemic *symptoms* such as fever, pain abdomen
and nausea, and local complaints such as severe eye pain, same side

headache and marked defective vision are constant symptoms. Eye shows ciliary congestion, hazy cornea, shallow A/C and dilated sluggish pupil. Vision is reduced to light perception. IOP is raised to approx 60 mm Hg (Normal is 10 to 21 mm Hg). The other eye has shallow A/C and narrow angle as seen by gonioscopy.

The final stage of any glaucoma is *absolute glaucoma*.

Management of acute congestive glaucoma is mainly three:

1. Drops such as pilocarpine or anti glaucoma drops such as Timolol (0.5%) twice a day. Pilocarpine may not act at higher ocular pressure.
2. Assisting reduction of IOP with *systemic* acetazolamide (250 mg 8 hrly; oral), intravenous urea or mannitol.
3. *Analgesics*–Sometimes even opioid derivative is used.

Local cortisone drops is applied to reduce inflammation. Whether IOP comes down or not, case is usually taken up for either laser iridotomy or for peripheral iridectomy in 48 hours. If angle is occluded by more than 1/3rd, then filtering surgery is needed.

Installation of miotics to contralateral eye should not be forgotten. Prophylactic laser iridotomy should be done in the contralateral eye also.

Nursing

1. The patient has such a severe pain that he needs all the comfort the nurse can give.
2. Nurse must see to it that (or even apply) the drops are applied as per instructions.
3. The excitement of the hospital atmosphere may precipitate an acute attack in the other eye. So the nurse must apply the miotic in the other eye.
4. She must gently tell the patient that surgery (or laser therapy) is the only permanent cure. At the same time she must strongly tell him that the surgery (or laser) is not for improving the sight.
5. She must have knowledge about glaucoma so that she can explain to the patient what he has.

OPEN ANGLE (CHRONIC SIMPLE) GLAUCOMA

This is met with in adults of more than 50 years of age. The angle and A/C are normal. The *cause* of obstruction to aqueous outflow is at trabecular meshwork (TMW). Its openings are reduced due to sclerosis and thus the aqueous out flow to Schlemm's canal is impaired. The IOP goes up (compare this situation with raised blood pressure due to sclerosis of blood vessel which reduces its lumen resulting in impairment to smooth flow of blood).

It is almost a *symptomless* disease. Patient may be change spectacles often – especially for reading. The eye is normal; so also angle by gonioscopy. Since there is no symptom and as patient is liable to loose his sight at the end, this is a dangerous eye disease.

The diagnosis depends on *three signs:*

a. *Raised intraocular pressure*—In the beginning it may not be present throughout the day and variation during the day is seen. If this variation is more than 8 mmHg it is suspicious (Fig. 6.h.9).

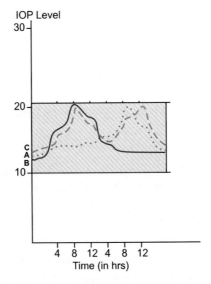

Figure 6.h.9: Diurnal variatiion in the early stage of glaucoma. A and B – Cases with once a day tension rise (monophasic). C – Case with rise in IOP twice a day (Biphasic rise)

Measurement of corneal thickness is necessary for correct assessment of IOP.

b. *Field of vision*—Scotoma (blind area) in the central 1/3rd of field of vision as well as constriction of peripheral field are seen. The central scotoma starts near blind spot and then spreads into a ring. This blind area spreads centrally towards fixation point and peripherally. The spread of scotoma continues in all direction. In the penultimate stage there is a seeing area around fixation point and a kidney shaped seeing area in the inferotemporal aspect of field. The rest of the field of vision is blind. The patient's acuity of vision remains the same as before almost unaffected upto this stage. So patient may not seek medical aid even at this stage. Finally the sight is lost.

c. *Optic disc changes*—The cup, the depression in the middle of the optic disc, which normally occupies the central 1/3rd of disc – enlarges. Finally the cup margin reaches almost the rim of disc. The colour of the optic disc also pales (Fig. 6.h.10). In the final stage the disc becomes papery white in colour (Glaucomatous optic atrophy).

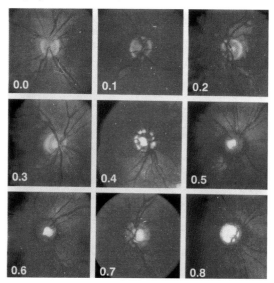

Figure 6.h.10: Optic disc in glaucoma. In normal cases the cup occupies 30% of the disc area (0.3). In early stage of glaucoma it occupies more than 50% of disc (0.5). In advanced case, cup reaches almost the edge of disc (0.8).

Gonioscopy reveals that the angle of anterior chamber is wide open (Figs 6.h.11 and 6.h.12).

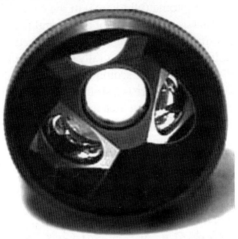

Figure 6.h.11: Three mirror gonioscope (goniolens)

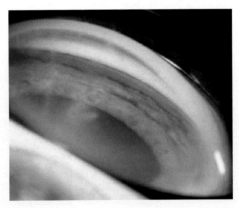

Figure 6.h.12: Gonioscopy view of angle of anterior chamber (A/C)

Management is mostly by *drugs, locally* which lower IOP (in various combinations and frequencies) with or without oral acetazolamide. To begin with one kind of drops is advised. If this is ineffective, it is changed to another drug rather than adding one more. After trying out single drug therapy in varying strength and frequencies, and if it fails, then only combination of drops is advocated.

The *drops used* are pilocarpine, adrenergic and prostaglandin analogues, and beta blockers. Some of the drugs used are: 1) Timolol (0.25 to 0.5%; bid). It is contraindicated in bronchial asthma. 2) Betaxolol (0.25% bid). This drug is safe in cardiopulmonary cases. 3) Cartelol (1% bid), 4) levobunolol (0.2% bid). The last mentiond drug is used once a day and 5) epinephrine (0.5% to 2%; used twice a day).

When medicines fail to control the ocular pressure and the disease is progressing, any one of the *filtering surgeries*–popular one is trabeculectomy–is done. In these operations a new communication is made between A/C and subconjunctival space (Compare it with treatment for hydrocephalus). The aqueous that is drained into subconjunctival space forms a bleb near the limbus.

Laser is also used to treat this condition. Argon laser trabeculoplasty (diode laser can be employed) opens the pores in TMW. Drainage devise is used in non responding cases (Fig. 6.h.13).

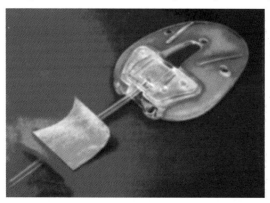

Figure 6.h.13: Drainage devise

Nursing

1. Since the drops therapy has to be tried to its utmost, the patient may have to be very patient and come for check up very frequently. The nurse has to encourage the patient so that he sticks to the instructions.
2. This may not be possible in India. So the nurse must get an idea of the patient's socio economic background. If this does not permit frequent visit to the hospital, she must bring it to the attention of the attending surgeon so that he can plan operation for the patient.

3. She must be capable of explaining to the patient the condition he has got.
4. When the patient is posted for surgery she must emphatically tell him that the surgery is NOT for improving the sight.

CERTAIN OTHER GLAUCOMAS

Following glaucomas are some of the *secondary glaucomas.*

Raised intra ocular pressure is seen in shallow chamber eye in which *lens has swollen up* (intumescent stage of cataract formation). Anterior dislocation of lens also is another cause. Management is by removing lens.

Dislocation of lens into anterior chamber (blocks anterior chamber angle), a pupil incarcerated lens and a posterior dislocated lens into vitreous (irritates ciliary body which results in increased aqueous secretion) can give rise to (secondary) glaucoma (Fig. 6.h.14).

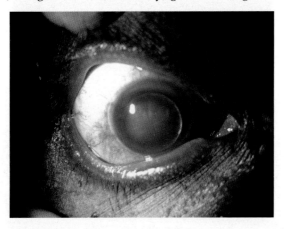

Figure 6.h.14: Subluxation of lens into A/C. It can cause raised IOP

Hyphema is blood in anterior chamber. It can be due to iridocyclitis (especially gonococcal or viral), trauma, postoperative and spontaneous (Fig. 6.h.15). It causes glaucoma. If intraocular pressure is raised, it can result in blood staining of cornea. This affects the central cornea with clear area all around (Fig. 6.h.16).

Hyphema mostly clears up well over months. Acetazolamide is given. Otherwise draining the blood by paracentesis is advised.

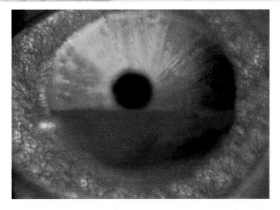

Figure 6.h.15: Blood in A/C (hyphema). It can cause glaucoma

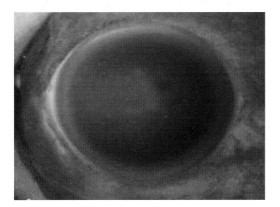

Figure 6.h.16: Blood staining of cornea due to hyphema

Raised IOP is seen with local use of steroids, after intraocular hemorrhage, along with uveitis, pseudoexfoliation of lens capsule (Glaucoma capsulare), aphakia and intra ocular tumors.

ABSOLUTE GLAUCOMA

It is the end stage of all glaucomas. The cornea is hazy, pupil dilated and fixed and iris is atrophic. IOP is raised to about 60 mm/Hg and optic disc shows glaucomatous optic atrophy (Fig. 6.h.17). Vision is totally lost. The eye is painful. The eye may finally become atrophic.

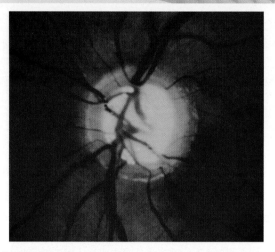

Figure 6.h.17: Advanced glaucoma cupping. The appearance of optic disc in an advanced glaucoma case. The disc is deep and pale

Management

It is mainly for the pain the patient has
1. *Destruction of ciliary body* is carried out to reduce IOP and to relieve pain.
2. *Retrobulbar alcohol* injection may be given (it should not enter the arterial circulation). It may be effective for 2 to 4 weeks in relieving pain.
3. *Enucleation* if pain is not relieved by the above methods.

(i) VITREOUS

Vitreous is a gel like structure situated in vitreous chamber behind the lens. It gives form to eye and is a source of nutrient to retina and lens.

VITREOUS OPACITIES

These opacities are divided into developmental and degenerative.
1. *Developmental:* These opacities are remnant of hyaloid system.

2. *Degenerative:* These can be–
   a. *Muscae Volitantes*—It is seen in elderly individuals. If seen against a bright background like clear sky, floaters of various shapes and sizes are seen. This needs no treatment. But sudden, marked increase in the number and size of floaters requires thorough study of fundus.
   b. *Synchisis scintilans*—In this condition cholesterol is deposited in the vitreous as multicoloured, glistening, gold dust like opacities floating in the fluid vitreous (Fig. 6.i.1). Any eye movement causes a "shower of gold particles" in vitreous. Except reassurance, treatment is not needed.

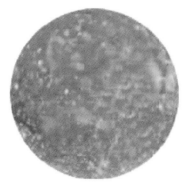

Figure 6.i.1: Synchisis scintilans

   c. *Asteroid hyalosis*—Spherical, white, calcium containing, fixed opacities are seen in vitreous (Fig. 6.i.2). It is met with in diabetics and hypercholesterolemia. Treatment is not needed.

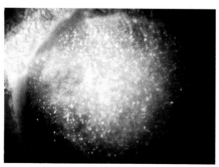

Figure 6.i.2: Asteroid hyalitis

d. *Other causes*—Hemorrhages into vitreous, inflammatory cells due to cyclitis and retinal vasculitis and neoplastic cells.

Nursing

1. In cases that have floaters in front of the eyes, the nurse must make all efforts to tell the patient that all is well.
2. At the same time, she should caution the patient that if there is any sudden increase in the number of floaters, he must attend the hospital immediately. But this caution should not make the patient "psychic".

VITREOUS HEMORRHAGE

Since it may cause sudden, painless loss of vision, it is an alarming condition for the patient. This loss may be preceded by floaters (spots in front of eye).

Causes

1. *Trauma*—It may be due to concussion or perforating injury. The bleeding is usually seen in vitreous.
2. *Ocular conditions*—Diabetic retinopathy, central retinal vein thrombosis (from the delicate new vessels), retinal neovascularisation, retinal tear (mostly in myopes) and rupture of intracranial aneurysm (subarachnoid hemorrhage) are some of the causes. Final picture is fibrous tissue proliferation in vitreous, retinal detachment, secondary glaucoma and blindness.

Management

1. Treatment of cause.
2. Bed rest with closure of eye (rest to the eye).
3. Closure of bleeding vessel by photocoagulation.
4. Vitrectomy if blood is not absorbed in 90-100 days.

SURGERY ON VITREOUS

The simplest surgical intervention is intravitreal injection of antibiotic or cortisone.

Vitrectomy

It is grouped into anterior vitrectomy, cone vitrectomy and total vitrectomy depending on the amount and position of vitreous that is to be removed. The entry is through pars plana.

The indications *for vitrectomy are–*

a. To remove blood in vitreous, tractional bands and membrane over retina
b. To treat abnormal retinal vessels
c. To deal with retinal breaks.
d. In endophthalmitis to remove the infected tissue.

(j) RETINA

A nurse need not know in detail about the retinal diseases. It is enough if she knows the basics of some of them.

Fundus can be examined with + 90 D lens using a slit lamp, with indirect or direct ophthalmoscope. The latter two methods have their own advantages and disadvantages.

Of special importance are disorders due to certain systemic diseases, retinal detachment, retinal dystrophy and tumor.

NORMAL FUNDUS

It has a pink colour. In the middle of retina is macula lutea. In the center of macula is fovea centralis. Three millimeter inside (medial or nasal) to retina's central point is the optic disc. It is an oval structure with a depression (cup) in its inner one third. The central retinal artery emerges from the cup and central retinal vein enters it to leave the eye. Peripherally retina ends at the ora serrata (Fig. 6.j.1).

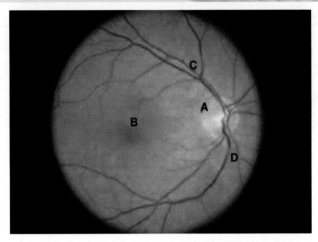

Figure 6.j.1: Normal ocular fundus. From the disc (A) emerges central retinal artery and into it enters the central retinal vein. They divide into upper (C) and lower (D) branches. The macula (B) is situated about 3 mm outside the disc

HYPERTENSIVE RETINOPATHY

Retinal vessels undergo changes like systemic vessels in hypertension. These changes in retina are divided into four *grades:*

Grade I: In this early stage there is narrowing of arterioles. Sclerosis is present in them.

Grade II: The narrowing increases. Changes appear where the arteries cross over the veins in ocular fundus – the veins are deflected at these A-V crossings.

Grade III: In the next stage the colour of arterioles resembles that of copper wire (and not red in colour). The blood gets stagnated in veins distal to A-V crossing with tapering of the veins on either side. Exudates along with hemorrhages are seen in the retina.

Grade IV: In the last stage the arterioles appear like fibrous thread (Silver wire appearance). Edema of optic disc appears (papilledema). This is more marked in *Malignant hypertension* in young patients (Fig. 6.j.2).

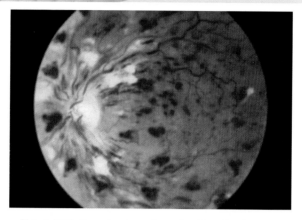

Figure 6.j.2: Hypertensive retinopathy. Vascular changes, hemorrhages and exudates are seen

PREGNANCY INDUCED HYPERTENSION

This is seen in eclampsia of pregnancy which occurs in late months of pregnancy. The retinal signs are marked narrowing of arterioles with exudates and hemorrhages. A-V crossing changes are not seen. These signs are met with when blood pressure goes above 180/110 mmHg and there is pedal edema. The appearance of retinal detachment is an indication for medical termination of pregnancy.

DIABETIC RETINOPATHY

The retinopathy due to diabetes depends on duration of systemic disease. The incidence is 7% in diabetic patients of 10 years duration and 63% for 15 years duration. The age at which the diabetes is detected also is important in the development and prognosis of retinopathy. It is basically a vascular occlusion.

The stages in the development of retinopathy are:

I. *Non Proliferative diabetic retinopathy (NPDR)*—The fundus picture ranges from very mild condition to very severe one. Microaneurysms and dot hemorrhages are seen. Both appear like red dots. Yellowish white exudates appear. They may surround the macular area (Fig. 6.j.3). Macula gets affected in this (and next) stage (Fig. 6.j.4).

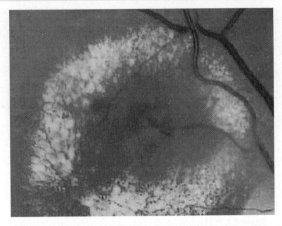

Figure 6.j.3: Diabetic retinopathy. Exudates are seen around the macula

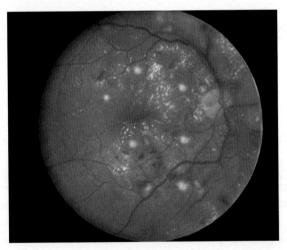

Figure 6.j.4: Diabetic retinopathy (Background stage). Hemorrhages and exudates are seen

II. *Proliferative diabetic retinopathy (PDR)*—It is usually seen when diabetes has lasted for about 20 to 30 years. Along with signs of NPDR, new vessels appear in the retina. Retinal and vitreous hemorrhage followed by fibrous tissue growth into vitreous occurs. Fibrous tissue and vitreous show contraction resulting in retinal detachment and many times blindness.

Management of diabetic retinopathy is mainly that of systemic disease.

1. Clofibrate helps in absorption of exudates. This drug has to be given for a long time.
2. Calcium dobesilate has beneficial effect.
3. Flavinoid group of drugs helps in treating capillary abnormality.
4. Aspirin may be effective.
5. Laser application to retina destroying portions of retina that are not functioning is the important treatment method. Either diode or Argon is used. Laser is not used in macular ischemic state.
6. In advanced cases surgery is undertaken for retinal detachment and vitreous hemorrhage (Vitrectomy).

RETINOPATHY OF PREMATURITY (RETROLENTAL FIBROPLASIA)

This is seen when premature infants of less than 33 weeks are weaned from the oxygen that was being given to them. The oxygen concentration in such a situation is more than 30%.

There is neovascularisation of retina especially beyond equator. There is proliferation and then contraction of the vascular tissue in the shunt area resulting in tractional retinal detachment and loss of vision.

Prevention is better.

Frequent observation is advised. Photocoagulation is recommended for progressive disease. In late stage vitrectomy and lensectomy are done; but the prognosis is poor.

Nursing

1. The nurse must be very careful while dealing with a premature baby. She must pay careful attention to the oxygen concentration.
2. In case this situation has occurred she must refer the baby to an ophthalmologist without fail.

RETINITIS PIGMENTOSA (RP)

It is degeneration of rods (and cones) of autoimmune etiology of retina starting at its middle region. It is a *hereditary disease.*

Its main *symptom* is *night blindness.* The vision is reduced by the associated cataract that is present. In the penultimate stage the field of vision is very much constricted so that the patient has *tubular vision.* At this stage the patient has difficulty in going about. The patient might go blind by 7th or 8th decade of life.

Examination of fundus shows a few floaters in *vitreous,* bone corpuscle like black *pigments* in the middle region of retina which are mostly around retinal veins. The retinal vessels are narrowed (Fig. 6.j.5). The optic disc and its nerve fibers slowly die (*consecutive optic atrophy*). The disc turns waxy yellow in colour. High percentage of myopia is met with. Ring shaped blind area (*scotoma*) occurs at the middle of field of vision. Later the scotoma spreads peripherally as well as centrally and in penultimate stage only a small seeing area is present around the fixation point *(tubular vision).*

RP has certain *variants* and some of them are *associated with* certain other problems such as glaucoma, deafness, hypogonadism, obesity, mental retardation, polydactyly and diabetes mellitus.

Treatment is ineffective. Genetic counseling should be given.

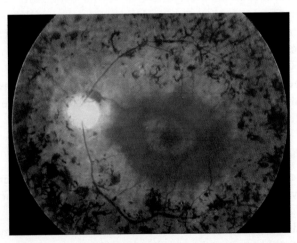

Figure 6.j.5: Fundus in retinitis pigmentosa. The bone corpuscles like pigments are seen in the mid periphery of the retina

Nursing

1. Tact must be shown by the nurse when mentioning about the prognosis. It should be told only to the closest relatives (father). This is to safe guard the future life of the patient. She should not tell many persons about the condition.
2. She must tell the same close relative that it is better that the patient marries out side his family (non consanguineous). This is a very difficult advice to follow in India.
3. More important is she must explain to the patient the difficulty he might encounter in dim light and with the reduced field of vision that might set in.

RETINAL DETACHMENT

It is separation of nine neuronal layers from pigment layer. It may be due to formation of hole or rupture in the retina through which fluid vitreous gets in. This results in retinal detachment (primary type). It can also be due to some fluid or solid (such as tumor behind the retina) pushing the retina away from choroid (secondary retinal detachment). Sometimes a fibrous tissue in the vitreous may pull on the retina causing detachment.

Symptoms

Flashes of light, change in the size of the objects seen and floaters in front of eye. Defective vision is met with when macula is involved or when there is vitreous hemorrhage. When these occur it may be sudden.

Signs

Visual *field* shows relative blind area (scotoma) which corresponds to detached area. *Intraocular pressure* is either reduced (usual) or raised (rare).

Fundus shows the detached retina to be gray in colour and thrown into folds. The vessels over the detachment appear smaller and darker (optical illusion). The hole or retinal break is red in colour (Fig. 6.j.6). The causative condition (in secondary type) is seen.

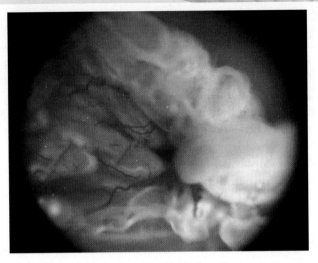

Figure 6.j.6: Retinal detachment. The tear in the retina is seen as red area. The detached retina has lost its pink colour and is thrown into folds

Management

Thorough examination is a pre requisite for a successful outcome. *Medical therapy* is not advised.

The aims of *surgical treatment* are to 1) close *all* the hole(s), 2) to bring the detached retina closer to choroid and 3) to drain any fluid under the retina. Closing the holes is achieved by cryo, laser or even by cautery.

RETINOBLASTOMA

It is a cancer derived from retina. In many, it is a hereditary disease. The hereditary cases are usually bilateral. Those which are non hereditary are commoner and are mostly unilateral.

Features

They are mostly seen within first two years of life. The pupil shows a white (actually yellow) reflex–so called leucocoria (*Amauratic cat's eye*). Sometimes squint and/or nystagmus may be present. Fundus shows the tumor mass which has a cheesy appearance and calcification. Retinal vessels course through and over it. Multiple tumor areas and retinal detachment are seen.

Later on the growth extends anteriorily and cause increase in intraocular pressure. Child has pain. If the tumor bursts through the sclera the ocular pressure comes down and pain is relieved. Sclera is the commonest site for perforation. When the tumor bursts through cornea, it is seen as fungating, bleeding mass.

Tumor extends via the optic nerve also. Finally the tumour spreads to regional lymph nodes, the cranial bones, distal bones, spinal cord, brain and, rarely, liver.

Its progress is divided into four stages.

Cases of retinoblastoma, if they survive, develop "second" cancer later in life.

Management

It is enucleation and/or radiotherapy. The method employed depends on so many factors.

Prognosis

Treated early, patient may survive. If it is in the final stage, death is almost inevitable.

Nursing

1. Lot of patience is required on the part of the nurse.
2. At any stage the nurse should not give too much of hope. She also need not tell about the "second" cancer to the parents of the patient.
3. Advice to get the eye removed (enucleation) is usually received with refusal. But the nurse must firmly tell about the possibility of the child dying later if the eye is not removed.

COMMOTIO RETINAE

It is otherwise known as *Berlin's edema*. It is caused by blunt injury to eye.

Patient *complains* of defective vision.

Signs include milky whitening of retina with cherry red spot at macula. Retinal vessels are normal (Fig. 6.j.7).

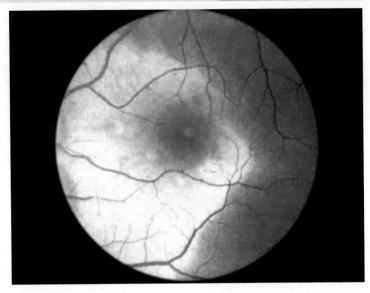

Figure 6.j.7: Commotio retina (Berlin's edema). The retina is white in colour due to fluid in it. The macula is cherry red in colour

Treatment: Not needed. Condition clears up spontaneously.

CENTRAL RETINAL VESSELS OCCLUSION

The central retinal artery (which supplies retina) or central retinal vein (which drains blood from retina) may get occluded. The vein gets occluded due to venous thrombosis, venous stasis or to pressure on vein by sclerotic retinal artery. The artery gets blocked due to embolism with or without central retinal artery spasm. The source of embolus is common carotid or heart valves.

It may be ischemic or non ischemic.

The patient gives history of marked defective vision (in venous occlusion) or even total loss of vision (in artery occlusion).

In venous block, *fundus* shows enormously engorged retinal veins with plenty of retinal hemorrhages and papilledema (Fig. 6.j.8). In arterial occlusion, narrowed arteries, cloudy white retina with cherry red spot at fovea are seen. In vein block intraocular pressure may go up.

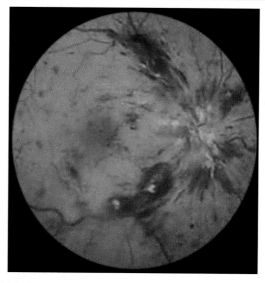

Figure 6.j.8: Central retinal vein occlusion. Shows plenty of hemorrhages. ("Angry looking fundus")

(k) OPTIC NERVE

Nurse need not know about diseases of optic nerve in detail. But she must have a basic knowledge of them.

PAPILLOEDEMA

It is a passive edema of optic disc (the nerve head) without any inflammation. It is usually bilateral; but edema may be of different degrees in the two eyes.

Causes

1. *Raised intracranial pressure*—Mostly due to tumors of brain, thrombosis of cavernous sinus, brain abscess, subarachnoid hemorrhage, aneurysm, hydrocephalus, meningitis and pseudotumour cerebri.

2. *Systemic causes*—Malignant hypertension, hypervitaminosis A, tetracycline, nalidixic acid, excess steroid, hypoparathyroidism and uremia.
3. *Orbital causes*—Tumours, inflammation.

Features—*Symptoms*, apart from that of causative lesion, are very minimal or even absent. Early morning headache is complained of. Transient blurring of vision may occur.

Fundus—Papilledema shows blurring of disc margin. Disc becomes more red and swells up. Veins are congested and dilated (Fig. 6.k.1). The edema subsides in all cases. But optic atrophy (Post papilledema) sets in. In this disc is grey in colour.

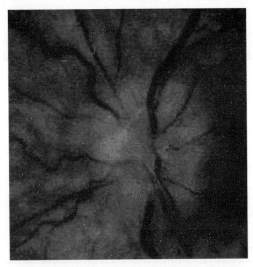

Figure 6.k.1: Papilledema–Disc margin is blurred and vessels are engorged

Management is that of cause. Edema disc can be brought down by decompression–making multiple slits in the optic nerve sheath.

OPTIC NEURITIS

It is inflammation of optic nerve. It may affect the optic disc (papillitis) or the portion of optic nerve behind the eye ball (retrobulbar neuritis). This latter condition can be acute or chronic.

Papillitis and acute retrobulbar neuritis are usually due to demyelinating diseases, infective causes or metabolic condition (such as diabetes). The chronic retrobulbar neuritis (otherwise known as toxic neuropathy) is due to takig of some poisonous material such as alcohol, tobacco, arsenic, chloroquine, etc.

The symptoms are sudden gross loss of vision (in papillitis and acute retrobulbar neuritis) or misty vision (toxic neuropathy). The signs are mainly that of fundus which are present only in papillitis. Field changes of different types are seen in these three conditions.

OPTIC ATROPHY

It is the disc condition when the optic nerve dies. The death is from retina to lateral geniculate body.

In total atrophy, pupil is dilated and fixed. In partial atrophy some vision is present with field defects (especially concentric contraction). The colour of the disc may not be an indication for extent of defective vision.

The optic atrophy may be primary (disc is white) (Fig. 6.k.2), glaucomatous (large cup with pale disc) (Fig. 6.k.3), secondary (pale disc with blurred margin) and consecutive (yellow disc) (Fig. 6.k.4).

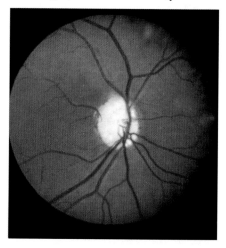

Figure 6.k.2: Primary optic atrophy. White disc on a normal fundus. Sometimes, even with this white disc acuity of vision may be normal

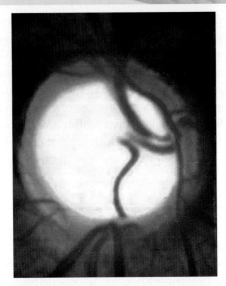

Figure 6.k.3: Glaucomatous optic atrophy showing the
white disc and markedly enlarged cup

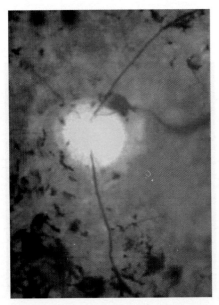

Figure 6.k.4: Consecutive optic atrophy in a case of retinitis pigmentosa.
The disc is yellow in colour

(I) SQUINT

It is also known as *strabismus* in which one eye is deviated relative to the other eye (Fig. 6.1.1).

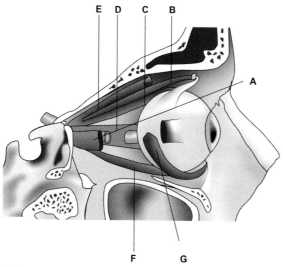

Figure 6.I.1: Extraocular muscles. A – Lateral rectus. B – Superior oblique. C – Superior rectus. D – Medical rectus. E – Levator palpebrae superioris (Not an extraocualr muscle). F – Inferior rectus. G – Inferior oblique

It is *divided into* paralytic (incomitant) and comitant squints. The former is due to paralysis of extra ocular muscle(s). Latter is due to some fault in the vision pathway caused by poor vision or to problem in brain in their ability to combine the images from the two eyes.

Table 6.I.1: Comparison between comitant and paralytic squints		
	Comitant squint	*Paralytic squint*
Onset	Gradual	Sudden
Cause	Poor vision or brain problem	Paralysis of extra ocular muscle(s)
Movements of eye	Present in all directions	Absent in one or more direction
Angle of squint	Same in all gaze/directions	Varies with eye movement
Diplopia	—	+
Systemic symptoms	—	Nausea and vertigo in the beginning

COMITANT SQUINT

This type of squint is caused by poor development of muscles outside the eye or due to defective vision since birth. They may be easily seen (called tropias) or the squint may be seen after some test (called phorias). The eye may deviate outside or inside. The former is common with short sight (myopia).

Symptoms are minimal except for cosmetic problem. The vision in squinting eye goes down.

PARALYTIC SQUINT

If there is a problem in nerves supplying the eye muscles or in the muscles themselves, it results in paralytic squint (Fig. 6.1.2).

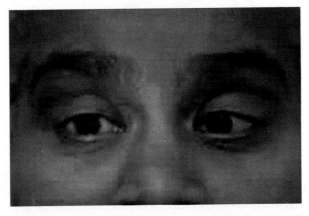

Figure 6.I.2: Case of convergent squint. Left eye is turned inwards, while the other eye is looking straight ahead

The chief *features are Diplopia* (double vision), *squint* and *head tilt* (Face turned).

Management

1. The *causative factor* must be dealt with.
2. Basically paralytic squint is mostly dealt by surgery while comitant squint is managed by non surgical methods. The surgery should be done when the patient is very young.

AMBLYOPIA

It is unilateral (sometimes bilateral) defective vision without any organic disease in the eye or in the visual pathway. The defective vision can be partial or total–the term *amaurosis* is used for the latter.

Nursing

1. The nurse must insist that any treatment that has to carried out (surgical or non surgical) must be done when the child is young (below the age of 8 or ten).
2. She must develop good relationship with the child so that the child develops confidence in the nurse. This is very important in the management of squint.
3. The nurse must closely interact with the orthoptist (the technician who treats squint cases).
4. The nurse must tell the parents that squint may spoil the chances of getting a job later in life by the patient.
5. Very important is that squint is considered as luck by many. If something bad happens to the family after the squint is corrected/treated, then the whole medical team will be blamed.

(m) REFRACTION

The subject of defective vision which can be corrected by spectacles (called refractive error) is not for a nurse. At the same time she should have some basic knowledge of these conditions since some of her patients (or their parents) may ask some doubts about them. These errors are checked by the procedure known as retinoscopy (Fig. 6.m.1) (in which trial set and trial frame are used) (Fig. 6.m.2). Nowadays autorefractometer is used (Fig. 6.m.3).

GENERAL

A normally developed eye acts as a convex lens with a power of + 60 D. The two major components producing this power are cornea (+ 43D) and lens (+17 D).

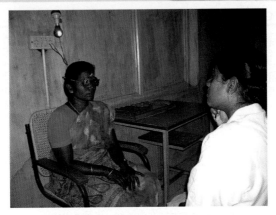

Figure 6.m.1: Retinoscopy procedure

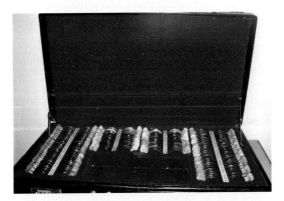

Figure 6.m.2: Trial Set

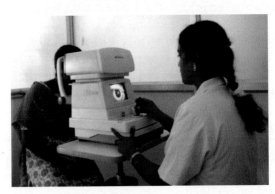

Figure 6.m.3: Auto refractometer

When a child is born, the length of eye ball is smaller. So a new born usually has a "defect". When the child grows up the length of eye ball increases so that by the age of 4 or 5 years it reaches the normal length of 24 mm.

In normal eye, the parallel rays of light are brought to a focus on the retina while eye is at rest. This state is known as *emmetropia*. If all parallel rays are not brought to a focus on the retina while eye is at rest then it is known as *ametropia*, i.e. patient has problem of seeing distance (and near) objects.

MAIN TYPES OF AMETROPIA

1. Myopia
2. Hypermetropia (Hyperopia) (Fig. 6.m.4)

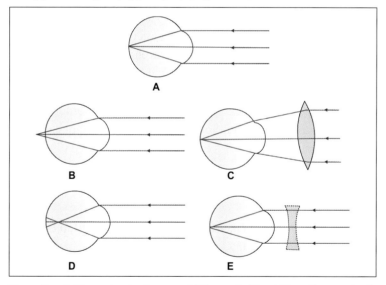

Figure 6.m.4: Figure showing the normal (A), myopic (B and C) and hypermetropic (D and E) eyes with the corrective lenses needed for the eyes with error

MAIN CAUSES OF AMETROPIA

1. *Axial*—All normal eyes have an axial length of about 24 mm. If there is any change in this length, it produces defect.

2. *Curvature*—If curvature of cornea (mostly) and lens is altered then ametropia occurs.

MYOPIA (SHORT SIGHT)

It is a condition in which the eye ball is longer or cornea is more curved.

There are three *varieties* of myopia:

Table 6.m.1: Varieties of myopia			
Features	*Simple*	*Congenital*	*Pathological*
Condition at birth	Normal	Large defect	Normal
Increase of error	Minimal	Minimal	Gross
Final Power	About-6D	Around–20D	Around–20 to 25D
Fundus Changes	Nil	Very minimal	Extensive

Symptoms: The patient has defective vision for distance. He will be comfortable with near vision work. In pathological myopia, some amount of "Night blindness" is present. If he develops cataract (especially in pathological myopia) the defect in vision worsens.
Signs: The eye looks larger. The anterior chamber is comparatively deep. Pupil is larger. In pathological myopia, visual field may show ring scotoma. The lens shows complicated cataract. In pathological myopia there are changes in the interior of the eye.

Treatment

1. Correction with spectacles—The minimum acceptable power should be prescribed.
2. Correction with contact lens.
3. Refractive surgeries which include radial keratotomy and LASIK (Figs 6.m.5 and 6.m.6).
4. Nutrition status must receive attention.
5. Genetic counseling should be given to patients with pathological myopia. Consanguineous marriage must be discouraged.

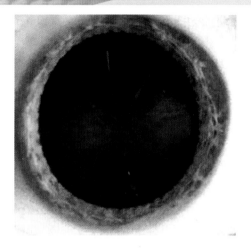

Figure 6.m.5: Radial keratotomy incisions in the peripheral cornea.
It corrects myopia

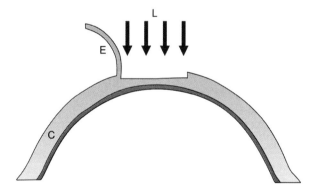

Figure 6.m.6: LASIK – Correcting refractive error with laser. L – Laser beam.
E – Corneal epithelium lifted up as a flap. C – Cornea

HYPERMETROPIA (HYPEROPIA)

It is that condition in which the eye is smaller in length or the cornea is less curved (very rare).

Symptoms are *eye strain* and *defective vision*. The defective vision is more for near vision (in mild cases), or it is present for both near and distance vision (cases with high error). Recurrent stye and lid margin inflammation may be complained of. Convergent squint is seen.

Signs include small eye and shallow anterior chamber. Fundus appearance may mimic that seen in brain tumors.

Treatment

1. Spectacles–Convex lens is recommended.
2. Contact lens.
3. Refractive surgeries which include LASIK.

PRESBYOPIA

If a person has to look at a near object (for practical purpose, within 33 cms) when his eye is already focused for a distance object, his eye undergoes *ACCOMMODATION*. In this the lens of the person becomes more convex.

When accommodation fails at the age of 40 and above due to hardening of lens or to weakness of ciliary muscle (caused by ageing), he is unable to see clearly small near objects, i.e. within 33 cms. This is known as *presbyopia*. It is a condition of failing near vision due to reduction in the accommodative capacity of the eye. This may set in *earlier* if the person is already hypermetropic, has general debility, develops early open angle glaucoma, has premature sclerosis of lens or he is doing excess near work, e.g. watch repairer.

The *symptom* is that of difficulty in focusing near objects such as in reading, writing, etc.

Treatment: Convex lens is advised.

LASIK

In this technique portion of cornea is excised with laser beam. This is useful for myopia as well as hypermetropia. Results are better if the defect is less than 8 Diopters (Spectacle power). It is performed in persons above the age of 21 years for whom there is no change of glasses power in a year. Lasik is not done in persons less than 20 years of age.

This is done as an out patient procedure. Sutures are not used. Complications are very infrequent. Glaring may be present for a few days. For some the original defect may return to some extent.

Nursing

1. The nurse is usually faced with questions about the refractive errors, the possibility of increase in the glasses power, whether it will occur in other family members and on LASIK.
2. The nurse must know that if the short sight defect is more than 6 diopter, there are possibility that the child will inherit it especially if the patient marries within the family members. She must be careful while explaining to the patient's relatives.
3. She must be able to answer questions on spectacles and contact lenses, and their maintenance.

7

Ophthalmic Surgeries and Nurses

ROLE OF NURSES IN EYE SURGERIES

The type of surgery performed can be grouped into three types:
1. *Regular:* These are the surgeries performed in main hospitals after admitting the patient.
2. *Ambulatory:* This is surgical patient care given under anaesthesia without actually admitting the patient overnight.
3. *Alternative:* This is the surgery that is performed in mobile hospitals such as military forward hospital or mobile eye hospital.

Basically the skill needed is the same in all these three types for a nurse except for minor differences.

MINOR SURGERIES

All cases posted for minor surgeries must sign the informed consent to protect the doctor and his team. If the patient is below 18 years, the signature must be obtained from a relative (In certain muslim countries such as Saudi Arabia, a female of whatever age cannot sign irrespective of whether the surgery is for herself or for a relative).

The *nurse's role* in minor surgeries is to prepare the patient, infuse courage into him, get ready the instruments and other materials, assist the surgeon during operation and to instruct the patient post operatively. The nurse must put the patient at ease before and after surgery. She must position the patient comfortably on the operation table.

MAJOR SURGERIES

The *needs* of a surgical patient can be broadly divided into physiological needs and psychological needs.

Physiological needs are the fluid balance (including electrolyte) of the patient (not of much importance in eye cases) and nutritional needs. It is important that the patient is in healthy condition.

In eye cases, nurse has important role to play. She must put courage into patient's mind. She must interact with the relatives, some of whom may need encouragement themselves. Their fears must be assuaged.

PREOPERATIVE NURSING CARE

- It is preferable that the bowel must be evacuated on the operation day. The head of patient must be covered by a cap. The male patients must shave their face (if there is no religious objection). The long hair of female patient is combed and plaited in two braids. They should be well tied so that the hair will remain in place for a few days.
- The nurse must check whether the basic *investigations* such as hemoglobin level, prothrombin time, creatinin level and blood sugar have been done. The blood pressure must be recorded. Any abnormality in them must be brought to the notice of the attending surgeon.
- The *eyelashes* (and sometimes the eye brows) are shaved. This practice is not followed in many centers nowadays.
- Any *source of infection* must be eliminated, especially lacrymal passage. The time honoured *"trial bandage"* method (trimming of eye lashes and applying bandage for 12 hours) is not practiced in most centers now. But preoperative conjunctival swabs for microbiological assessment and use of antibiotic drug to eye must be carried out.
- The *face* is well scrubbed and cleaned with sterile cotton.
- Just before going for operation, skin around the eye should be cleaned with 10% povidone iodine pyrolidone and the conjunctival sac irrigated with 5% povidone iodine. Proper draping which covers even the eye lashes is important during operation.
- The eye to be operated is marked with a marker pen with an 'X' mark. The eyes are covered with sterile gauze so that the patient may not put his unsterile finger on it.
- The patient puts on clean gown. Jewellery, removable prosthesis, wigs and dentures are removed.
- The nurse must instruct the patient about anaesthetic procedure and about the operation itself. She must encourage the patient and allay his fears—fear of unknown, of anaesthesia and of operation. If the patient is apprehensive or emotional, it upsets operation.

- Any preoperative drug that has been ordered should be given.
- The identification tag must be checked and the necessary materials that are needed in the operation theatre for him (such as IOL) must be sent along with the patient. He must be handed over to the OT in charge.
- The patient must be sent in time to OT

PERIOPERATIVE NURSING CARE

A nurse must have a general idea about the operation theatre (Fig. 7.1).

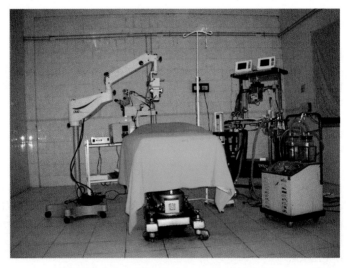

Figure 7.1: Appearance of an eye operation theatre

Theatre (OT): Planning and construction are very important. Many places have their OT lined with stainless steel. Electrical points should be "buried". There should be three "barricades" between OT and the outside world. Outside air should never enter OT without purification. Air should be cleaned by use of laminar flow. Filters should be fitted in air conditioners. Rotating ultra violet light is to be employed before and in between operations. Formaline fumigation using formaldehyde (Formaldehyde + water in 1%) in container left for 4 hours purifies OT air. Formaldehyde tablets are also used. OT is cleaned daily. Washing the OT floor with chlorhexidine or lysol weekly and monthly is done. Microbiological culture is done once in 3 months. The accepted level is 20 colonies and two colonies for bacteria and fungi respectively.

Sterility level of various items that come in contact is divided into:

a. *Critical*—These are items that come into contact with open body tissues.
b. *Semicritical*—Those that come in contact with intact skin or mucous membrane in the operating field. These are sterilized immediately before surgery.
c. Non *critical*—Those items that come in contact with skin or mucous menbrane remote from operating field.

Basic Principles of Sterile Technique

a. Sterile items are used within sterile field—These include drapes, sponges and instruments. If materials are unused earlier, it must be flash autoclaved before surgery. Materials in this area should not go to unsterile field. Unsterile materials and persons should not enter sterile field.
b. Sterile persons should never touch unsterile area or materials. They must keep within the sterile area. OT floor is the most unsterile area.
c. Persons should be gowned and gloved. The gown is considered sterile only in the upper half of front portion and from elbow to gloves. The sterile hand should never be lowered below the waist.
d. Sterile field must be always in view of the scrub nurse.
e. Operating tables are sterile only on top; but never on the sides (even when draped) or the underside.
f. Micro organisms must be kept to the minimum. This is done by washing, by antiseptic methods and sterilisation. The personnel and patient must be as clean as possible. Hair of patient and personnel must be covered. Some areas of patient such as his intestines may have lot of microorganism. It is accepted that microorganisms cannot be totally eliminated. But they should be kept at very minimum.

During perioperative time (i.e. during surgery) the patient is taken care of by *perioperative team*. This team is grouped into non sterile team and sterile team. The former group includes anaesthetist, anaesthetic assistant, circulating nurse, theatre assistant, patient transporting team and students. The sterile team consists of surgeon, first assistant and scrub nurse.

It should be remembered that in most of the eye surgeries, the nurse has not much part to play in the operation field. Either the surgeon does the surgery all alone or his doctor assistant helps him. But when the nurse is called in, she has to be alert, intelligent and useful.

The *nurse in OT* may be the one who is in the field of operation (*scrub nurse*) or the one who is around in the operation theatre (OT) getting the sterile materials to the operation area (*circulating nurse*).

Duties of Scrub Nurse

She must have a good knowledge of the operation procedure and the instruments. It will be ideal if she is *ambidextrous*, i.e. ability to use both the hands equally well. The simplest way to start acquiring this skill is to brush the teeth with the left hand (by a right handed person) and then to practice use of scissors, suturing and suture cutting with the left hand.

- She has to put the patient on the table in the correct position especially for the operating microscope.
- She has to get the microscope ready–fixing of sterile cups and the sterile drape over the eye pieces, and focusing the microscope.
- She has to clean the patient's face especially around the eye to be operated and drape the case.
- Handling instruments. This requires a good knowledge about instruments and the way to handle them. She must know when to hand over certain instruments and how to hand over them. For example she must know how to hand over a blade (blunt side towards the surgeon) or a forceps.
- She may have to manage the bleeding either by irrigation or by sponging.
- Most of the surgeons do the suture cutting themselves. But when necessary the scrub nurse may have to do this. She must

employ the tri pod grip technique and keep the scissors parallel to tissues near the suture. In eye operations, most of the sutures are cut close.

- In phaco surgery, her help is needed with the phaco machine. For this the nurse must have very good knowledge about phaco machine and its working.
- In *antiglaucoma* surgeries, the scrub nurse has minimal role to play.
- In *corneal grafting*, the scrub nurse has to get ready the donor corneal tissue and help in cutting the disc to be transplanted. She must know the details of the donor and the nature and time of his death.

Duties of Circulating Nurse

- She must have thorough knowledge about the case that is being operated upon. She must be able to provide the surgeon any preoperative details he might require. She must see to it that the correct surgery is being done for correct eye.
- She must coordinate the activities of all the persons inside the OT. She must be the link in the communication between the various staff inside the OT.
- She must see to it that the necessary instruments are handed over to the sterile team in time and in sterile condition. She must know how to hand over in sterile condition the sterile items to the sterile field.
- She must be able to identify any change in the general condition of the patient.
- She must have the capacity to teach the students (medical and nursing) about OT—maintenance, sterilisation procedure, patient preparation and even about the operation.

Draping is done with linen (danger of infection present if it gets wet), muslin or paper.
- Drape should be limited within the operation field.
- Once applied the drape should not be moved.
- Discard the drape if it touches the floor or has a hole in it.

- Do not flourish the drape.
- The gloved hands should not touch the patient's skin.
- An eye drape usually is about 3' in length and about 1 ½ feet in breadth. The central hole (for eye) is about 4" x 4".

Preparations

Personnel—It involves wearing clean OT dress, washing and scrubbing of hand and forearm and putting on sterile gloves. *Scrubbing* methods differ between centers. Cap and mask must be worn before scrubbing. The hands and forearm (upto just below elbow) are rinsed with warm water first. Then antiseptic soap is applied for 3 to 5 minutes for each hand and forearm, or 20 strokes for hands, fingers and forearms. Hands and wrist are scrubbed first. Forearms are scrubbed upto 2 inches below elbow after this. In some centers sterile brush is used after applying antiseptic soap; in other centers brush is not used. Instead of antiseptic soap, betadine solution (with or without brushing) is used for 5 minutes to clean the hand and forearm. Hands are then washed with sterile water. While washing the hands should never be held below the level of elbow. Once scrubbed the hands and forearms should not be lowered below the waist. After scrubbing, drying with towel must be started with hand and then go upto wrist and finally the forearm. It should NEVER be in the reverse order.

The *gown* is worn without touching the outer (working) surface with the washed hands. Water should not drip over the gown. Both scrub nurse and circulating nurse must know how to gown themselves. They also must learn how to gown others.

A gowned sterile person must cross another such gowned person 'back-to-back' only, so that their sterile gloved hands may not become unsterile. Once gowned the arms should never be folded with hands in the axilla.

Use of *gloves* is the rule now. (About two decades ago many eye surgeons in India used to operate with bare hands. Infection was infrequent then also !). The nurse must know the correct way of putting on gloves. Wearing of gloves is done in *two ways*:- a) In closed gloving technique, the gloves are handled and worn by the scrub nurse with her hand covered by the sleeve of gown. b) In open gloving method, the gloves are worn with the sterile hand which is outside the sleeve of the gown. In the latter methods she should not touch the working surface of the glove with her sterile fingers. A nurse must practice and be expert in these two methods. She also must be good in gloving another

Instruments—The sterile instruments are laid on the *tray*. The scrub nurse must do preparation of the tray in the sterile field of OT after she has scrubbed and worn sterile dress. The instrument tray (or table) must be already wiped clean. Scrub nurse spreads sterile towel over it. The instruments are laid on this towel in the order in which they will be needed during surgery. The towel should never get wet during operation. Cotton tipped applicator, cellulose sponge or spear is used to absorb fluid during operation. These can be sterilised along with instruments.

Sterile items can be opened by peel back method or hand held method of distribution. The nurse must master these two techniques.

At the end of the operation, the instruments are to be cleaned. Disposable sharp instruments and other disposable items are discarded separately. Ophthalmic instruments are delicate ones. Gentle handling is needed. The clotted blood, tissues and fluids must be cleaned well with soft tooth brush. This is important with instruments like forceps and instruments with hinges such as needle holder. The joints of the instruments should be specially cleaned. Ulrasonic cleaners are very useful in this respect. Water is enough to clean. After every cleaning process the instruments must be lubricated to protect against deposits and impurities. After cleaning, the instruments are packed and sent for sterilisation. The nurse should be cautious so that she herself does not get infected. Gloves and protective goggles must be worn.

It should be remembered that cleaning of instruments starts with scrub nurse. She removes the blood and tissues from the instruments as soon as she gets them back from the surgeon. Later these instruments are packed and taken to *OT processing room* where it is cleaned and dried. Final cleaning (if needed) and sterilisation take place in the *clean processing room*.

The most important part of the nursing is in the immediate post operative period.

Postoperative Period

- If the surgery has been done under general anaesthesia, the nurse has to stand by to help the anaesthetist. Once the patient recovers fully from anaesthesia (regional or general) she has to assure the patient that all is well.
- Some patients may be agitated–especially cataract cases for whom eye patching is not done. She must see that the patient does not meddle with his operated eye.
- The case sheet must be checked for the entry of details of operation and of proper postoperative instructions. The case should be properly transferred to ward (usually 30 minutes after surgery) through a responsible person along with case sheet.
- The post operative instructions must be scrupulously followed.
- During the immediate postoperative period, if the nurse feels that there is something wrong or if patient is restless or coughs, she must immediately send for the surgeon.
- Mouth care must be given. Evacuation of bowel should be attended to. She should watch out for urinary retention.
- Early ambulance is better. Too much sedation should not be given so as to avoid the problem of "striking the bandage".
  Dressing of the operated eye is done daily.
  Equipments needed (for dressing)–
1. Clean trolley with a sterile tray covered with sterile cloth.
2. Sterile cotton balls or spears.
3. Medications–Antibiotic, cortisone and mydriatic drops.
4. Anaesthetic eye drops.
5. Sterile patch (pad) and paper plaster.
6. Kidney tray.
7. Torch light and loupe.
8. Distance vision chart.
    - Some surgeons do the first dressing after the surgery at the slit lamp. If this be the case, slit lamp must be kept ready and clean by the nurse.

- The postoperative patients must have some diversion/ recreation. Light may be uncomfortable, and music is ideal.
- The room should be neat and ventilated. The patient should be up and about as early as possible.
- At the time of discharge, the vision (with glasses, if needed) must be checked and recorded.
- The patient must be told about the medications (frequency, dose, method of applying) and the toxic symptoms for which he should seek immediate attention.
  - He must be instructed about the type of work and way of life he must follow and when to start these.
  - He must be informed about his follow-up visits. He must have the emergency number of the hospital.

CHAPTER

8

Ocular Surgeries and Anaesthesia

I. GENERAL ANAESTHESIA

It is usually not needed for most of the eye surgeries. It is mainly *indicated in* 1) operations of long duration, 2) children, 3) apprehensive patients, 4) patients who specifically desire it, 5) injuries especially with open globe, and for 6) patients who are sensitive to local anaesthetic drugs.

While giving general anaesthesia it should be remembered that 1) there should be good relaxation of muscles, 2) it should lower the ocular pressure (IOP), 3) there should not be any retching during intubation or nausea/vomiting during recovery period.

General anaesthesia usually reduces *IOP*. But agents like trichlorethylene and ketamine increase IOP. Halothane produces reduction in IOP. Hypnotics, barbiturates and tranquilisers cause reduction in IOP. But oral chloral hydrate solution does not affect IOP. Reduction in IOP is desirable in eye operations.

General anaesthetic agents can be inhalation (nitrous oxide, halothane, isoflurane and desflurane) and intravenous (Thiopental, ketamine, fentanyl, diazepam and midaxolam).

II. REGIONAL ANAESTHESIA

This is the method for most of the eye operations. The eye should be anaesthetic, devoid of movements (akinesia) and the lids should not close.

1. *Retrobulbar* (ciliary block)—To anaesthetise the interior of the eye. About 1.5 ml of lignocaine (2%) mixed with adrenaline and hyalase is injected behind the eyeball.
   Peribulbar block—The local anaesthetic agent is injected around the globe. Facial block is not needed with this method.
2. *Facial nerve block*—This paralyses the seventh cranial (facial) nerve so that closure of lids is temporarily abolished (Fig. 8.1).
   Advantages of regional anaesthesia:
   a. Lesser postoperative retching and pain.
   b. Patient is conscious during surgery.
   c. No complication that is seen with GA.
   d. Oculocardiac reflex is abolished.

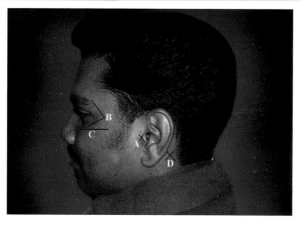

Figure 8.1: Methods of facial block. A – O' brien.
B – Von Lint. C – Atkinson. D – Nabath

3. *Local drops*—One drop of 4% lignocaine is instilled once a minute for five times. This produces enough anaesthesia to perform any eye surgery–intraocular and of conjunctiva. It lasts for about 15 minutes. Lack of akinesia is the main problem.

LOCAL ANAESTHETIC AGENTS

They are amino ester agents such as cocaine, procaine (0.5 to 2 %), tetracaine (1 to 2 %), or amino amides agents such as lidocaine (lignocaine 0.5 to 2 %) or xylocaine (2 to 4%), bupivacaine (marcaine 0.25 to 0.5 %) and mepivacaine (0.5 to 2 %). The duration of action ranges from 60 minutes to 10 hours.

Adverse Effects

1. *Allergy*: Mostly seen with ester-linked group. This is due to its breakdown product, para amino benzoic acid. Sometimes the preservative used in it such as sodium metabisulphite might be the cause.
2. *Tissue toxicity* especially of nerves and muscles occur in high concentration.
3. *Systemic toxicity* mainly affecting cardiovascular and central nervous systems.

4. *Neurotoxicity*: This is seen mostly with ester-linked agents. It is more if sodium metabisulphite is added to an agent with low pH. The nerve can be damaged by the needle or pressure ischemia if intraneural injection is made. This is not of great importance in ophthalmology.

5. Of greater importance is *myotoxicity* which is seen in higher concentration. This may affect the extraocular muscles leading to even permanent paralysis.

ADJUVANTS

1. *Adrenaline:* Sometimes drugs such as adrenaline and/or hyaluronidase are mixed with the local anaesthetic agent. Adrenaline delays absorption and increases duration of action of anaesthetic agent.

2. *Hyaluronidase:* It spreads the injected agent across connective tissue barrier.

A. MINOR SURGERIES

1. Foreign Body Removal

Equipments needed (Fig. 8.2):

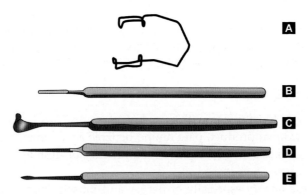

Figure 8.2: Instruments for removal of foreign body from conjunctiva and cornea. A – Barraquer eye speculum. B – Nicati foreign body spud. C – Desmarre's lid retractor. D – von Graefe's cataract knife. E – Foreign body needle

1. Slit lamp – Should be well cleaned.
2. Sterile tray containing foreign body spud, 24G needle, cotton balls and patch (eye pad).
3. Lignocaine (2%) drops.
4. Sterile fluorescein (2%). This is rarely required and that too only in corneal foreign body removal.
5. Paper plaster.
6. Antibiotics, homatropine and cyclopentolate eyedrops.
7. Dastoor lid retractor or wire speculum.

Foreign body removal from conjunctiva and cornea is done usually as outpatient procedure under slit lamp. It is done after local application of anaesthetic agent.

Nursing

• The nurse must explain to the patient what is going to be done. Although the foreign body itself causes so much of irritation and even agony, most of the patients accept this calmly. More patience is required with children. Infants may sometimes need short anaesthetic.
• The patient has to be seated at the slit lamp by the nurse and chin and forehead of patient properly positioned at slit lamp.
• Conjunctival foreign body is usually removed with a cotton swab or with a needle.
• Corneal foreign body in its superficial layers is removed with a spud or with a 24G needle.
• After removal of foreign body, antibiotic drop is applied and patient is advised to apply the same hourly. If it had been corneal foreign body, application of cyclopentolate or homatropine locally after removal is optional. It should be applied only at the doctor's instruction. Atropine should never be applied as it keeps the pupil dilated for 7 to 10 days causing glaring and discomfort.
• It is better that the foreign body that was removed is shown to the patient.
• Nurse must advise about the drops application at home, the method and about the review next day.

Deeply imbedded corneal foreign body should be removed only in operation theatre. Non reactive, multiple corneal foreign bodies are sometimes not removed.

If foreign body is in superior fornix, double eversion of upper lid is needed and is done with the help of Dastoor's lid retractor.

2. Chalazion Surgery

The surgery is known as incision and curettage (Fig. 8.3).

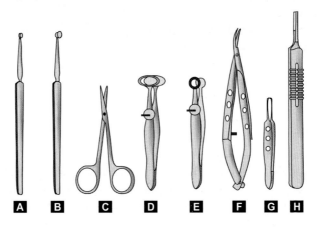

Figure 8.3: Tray for Chalazion surgery. A and B – Chalazion scoop. C – Straight scissors. D and E – Chalazion clamp. F – Curved scissors. G – Forceps. H – Bard Parker handle

Equipments needed-
1. *Instruments*—Chalazion clamp, Bard Parker or cataract knife, chalazion scoop, fine toothed forceps, fine scissors.
2. Lignocaine (2%). About 2 cc of it is loaded in a syringe to which a 24 G needle is attached.
3. Lignocaine (2%) drops.
4. Antibiotic drops, drape, sterile cotton balls, patch and paper plaster.

Nursing

- The nurse cleanses the skin of lids and surrounding area with betadine and irrigates the conjunctival sac with betadine. The eye area is draped with sterile drape.
- Local anaesthesia (lignocaine) is given usually by the surgeon and rarely by the nurse. The local infiltration is given in a V

shaped manner on the skin aspect with the apex away from lid margin and the arms of V enclosing the lesion. After anaesthetic injection, the patient should not be left alone by the nurse.

- Lignocaine (2%) is applied twice at one minute interval in the conjunctiva.

The surgery consists of vertical incision over the conjunctiva, scooping out the contents of chalazion and finally removing the capsule.

Once the surgery is over, the chalazion clamp is removed and immediately the lids are closed.

- The nurse places a patch over the closed lids and gently applies pressure over the closed lids for about 5 minutes. This stops the bleeding from operated site. The lids are opened, antibiotic ointment applied and a firm patch is applied. This can be removed after 2 hours. After this, frequent application of drops is recommended.
- Pain reliever may be taken. The patient comes the next day for review.
- If the patient gives history of recurrent attacks of chalazion, the nurse must insist that the patient gets his blood sugar checked (older patients) and his eyes checked for glasses. The patient also must take a course of systemic broad spectrum antibiotic.

3. Pterygium Surgery

The operative treatment for pterygium is many and varied. It may be:

1. Simple release of pterygium and its excision (Bare sclera method).
2. Releasing the pterygium and burying its apex under the adjacent conjunctiva.
3. Excising the released portion of pterygium and covering the raw area with materials such as conjunctiva

Agents such as mitomycin C are sometimes used locally in recurrent cases.

Equipments needed (Fig. 8.4):

1. *Instruments:* Speculum, conjunctival forceps, colubri forceps, fine knife or cataract knife, Took's corneal splitter, conjunctival scissors and needle holder.

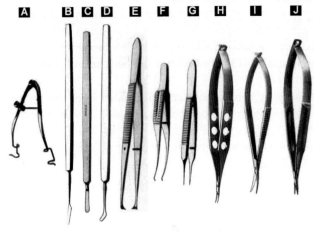

Figure 8.4: Pterygium operation instruments. A – Clark speculum. B – Anderson pterygium knife. C – Took's corneal splitter. D – Paton's corneal dissector. E – Graefe fixation forceps. F – Barraquer colibri forceps. G – Castroviejo suture forceps. H – Sinsky tying forceps. I – Castroviejo corneal scissors. J – Heiss needle holder

2. Suture—Perlon (11/0).
3. Lignocaine (2%)—Injectable and drops.
4. Antibiotic eye drops, drapes, swabs as buds or as spears (Fig. 8.5), patch and paper plaster.
5. Mitomycin C drops.

Nursing

- The nurse must explain that the procedure, although a "minor" one, can be considered "major" as the cornea is dissected. She must tell this before the patient is got ready for surgery.

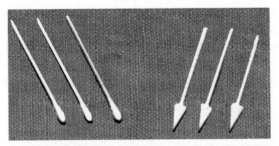

Figure 8.5: Cotton buds and spears. These are used instead of cotton balls during eye surgeries

- She also has to tell the patient in as gentle a manner as possible that there is a possibility of recurrence.
- After operation, it is preferable to apply a patch which can be removed the next day. After this antibiotic drops (4 times a day) is applied for about a week.

  (In some centers, dacryocystectomy and dacryocystorhinostomy are done in the major OT)

B. MAJOR SURGERIES

Following are some major eye surgeries. A nurse must be familiar with the steps of these common operations so that she may be of real use in the operation theatre and may be able to explain in a better way to the patients what is going to be done for him.

It must be remembered that there are so many modifications in any surgery and each surgeon has his own way of operating.

It should be again emphasized that any case posted for operation under regional anaesthesia must be prepared for conversion to general anaesthesia.

1. Cataract

This is usually done under local anaesthesia – Ciliary and facial blocks (or) peribulbar block. Locally 2% lignocaine drops are instilled.

The introduction of operating microscope, phaco machine (which divides the lens nucleus into small fragments) and automated continuous irrigation-aspiration system has brought in much improvement in the cataract surgery (Fig. 8.6).

1. *Extracapsular cataract extraction (ECCE)*—In this technique the nucleus, cortex and central part of the anterior capsule only are removed. Posterior capsule and peripheral portion of the anterior capsule are left behind in the eye at the end of surgery. This method is used especially if posterior chamber IOL implantation is planned since an intact posterior capsule is needed to support the IOL and to prevent it from slipping into vitreous (Figs 8.7i to xiii).

   The superior rectus suture is applied (not mandatory). The conjunctiva is cut at limbus in the upper quadrant and reflected back. Bleeding points secured. Anterior chamber is entered with

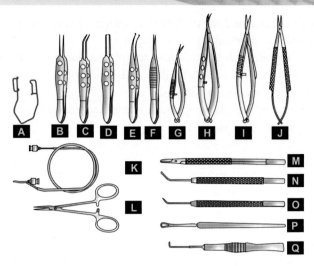

Figure 8.6: A few of the instruments used for cataract operation. A – Barraquer wire speculum. B – Jaffee tying forceps (straight). C – Mc Pherson forceps; angled, D – McPherson corneal forceps. E – Arruga capsule forceps. F – Wills hospital utility forceps. G – Vannas capsulotomy scissors (angled). H – Castroviejo corneal scissors (universal). I – Westcott tenotomy scissors. J – Barraquer micro needle holding forceps. K – Simcoe I/A canula (Direct). L – Hartman straight mosquito forceps. M – Castroviejo blade breaker. N – Nightingale capsule polisher. O – Sinskey II lens manipulating hook. P – Lewis lens loop (small). Q – Smith lens expressor

the tip of blade at limbus. Viscoelastic is injected into anterior chamber. The anterior capsule of lens is cut open in a circular fashion with the help of bent 24 G needle (Or it can be peeled off in a circular fasion). The limbal incision is extended to a length of 3 mm to 5.2 mm (or, the incision is made away from limbus in sclera and tunneled into anterior chamber). The cut circular anterior capsule piece removed. The rest of capsule is separated from the cortex by irrigating with fluid (hydrodissection). The nucleus is divided into pieces with phaco and aspirated out. The cortex that remains is also aspirated out. (Or, the nucleus can be expressed out with pressure and counter pressure and the remaining cortex aspirated out). Making a hole in the iris is not needed. The IOL is introduced behind the iris. The haptics (limbs) of the IOL are usually between the peripheral portion of anterior capsule and the posterior capsule. The haptics should

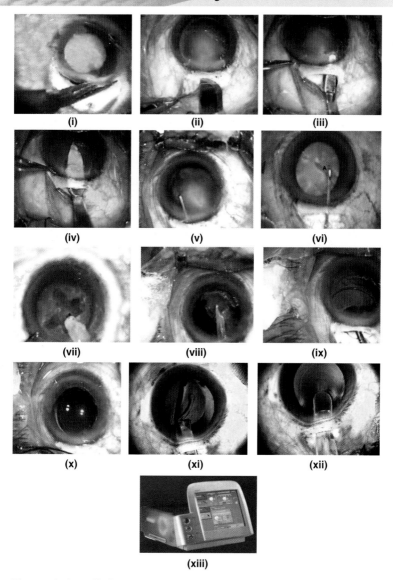

Figures 8.7i to xiii: Steps of cataract surgery. (i) Limbal opening. (ii) (Alternate) frown incision made near limbus. (iii) Beginning of incision into A/C. (iv) Incision completed. (v) Capsulotomy (opening into anterior capsule) with needle. (vi) Anterior capsule (A) peeled off in circular pattern. (vii) Nucleus divided by phaco machine. (viii) Cortex aspirated. (ix) IOL inserted into A/C. (x) IOL in position in the bag (between anterior and posterior capsules). (xi) (Another case) Foldable IOL being inserted into A/C. (xii) The IOL unfolding itself in the bag. (xiii) Phaco machine

be in horizontal position. The limbal wound is closed with 10/0 suture. With the advent of rollable or foldable IOL, the size of the (limbal) incision has come down to one mm. (There are so many modifications in ECCE). (For details of IOL – See under "Lens")

2. *Intracapsular cataract extraction (ICCE)*—In this type of operation, the lens is removed completely. Nowadays it is not done as frequently as it was done about 20 years ago (Figs 8.8i and ii).

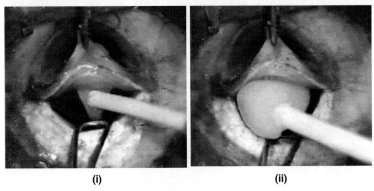

(i)　　　　　　　　　(ii)

Figure 8.8: Removal of cataract with cryo equipment. (i) Frozen cryo tip placed on the lens. The lens gets stuck to the cryo tip; (ii) The lens which is attached to the cryo tip due to the ice that has formed is being removed in toto

After superior rectus suture application, a limbal based conjunctival flap is reflected. Limbus is opened for 120° and a peripheral iridectomy done. The lens is removed in toto by cryo (Fig. 8.9). The lens can also be removed by using intracapsular forceps, vectis (in subluxated lens) or by erysiphake. In hypermature cataract, tapping at 6 O'clock position with counter pressure at 12 O'clock position expresses out the lens (Smith – Indian method). Limbal wound is closed with 10/0 suture. The conjunctival wound closed with continuous suture.

Complications

I. Complications of anaesthesia:
 1. Reaction to drug.
 2. Retrobulbar hemorrhage (does not occur with peribulbar block). Operation should be postponed by ten days.
 3. Perforation of globe while giving the injection.

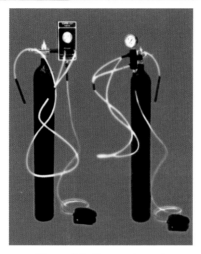

Figure 8.9: Cryo equipment

II. Operative–
1. Expulsive hemorrhage.
2. Vitreous loss (in ICCE).
3. Capsular rupture (in planned ECCE).

III. Post operative–
1. *Iris prolapse*—Not seen with modern day technique.
2. *Shallow chamber*—Due to wound leak, pupillary block or cilio choroidal detachment.
3. *Retinal detachment*—Seen in cases with retinal degeneration as in high myopia and in cases that had vitreous loss. This is common with ICCE.
4. *Corneal edema*—It is due to corneal endothelial damage caused during surgery or later by vitreous touching back of cornea. An A/C IOL can also cause corneal damage and corneal edema.
5. *After cataract*—Commonly seen after ECCE.
6. Infection.

IV. Complications associated with IOL–
1. *Malposition of IOL*—It may be decentered (this is mostly due to faulty technique), or may move up or down due to subluxation.

2. *Corneal endothelial damage*—More common with A/C IOL.
3. Dislocation of IOL into vitreous.
4. *Swinging of IOL*—Seen with small IOL with haptics placed vertically.

2. Glaucoma

In glaucoma the aqueous humor is not able to go out by the normal outlet due to block at or near the angle of A/C. So a new artificial route should be created. This new route may connect the anterior chamber with space under the conjunctiva, or it may connect the anterior chamber to the space between sclera and choroid.

The surgeries for glaucoma can be *grouped into*—

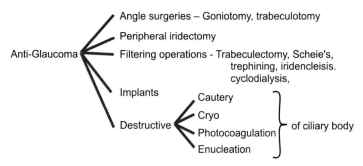

(Enucleation is done for absolute glaucoma cases that have pain which cannot be relieved).

Peripheral Iridectomy

In glaucoma cases, iridectomy (excising a small piece of iris) is done as a curative procedure for narrow angle glaucoma (in its first three stages) and along with other antiglaucoma (filtering) operations.

In this surgery, after keeping the eye open with speculum, conjunctiva is cut at the limbus for 4 mm and pushed back. A small incision is made at limbus. Peripheral iris usually comes out through the limbal opening (or is made to come out). A bit of iris tissue is cut from the peripheral portion of it that has come out. Limbal wound may be closed with a single 10/0 suture. There is no need to close the conjunctival wound (Fig. 8.10).

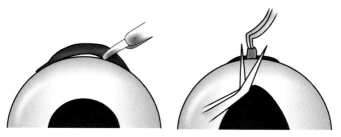

Figure 8.10: Steps of peripheral iridectomy. A – Limbal incision.
B – Cutting of peripheral iris

Filtering operations are those in which an artificial, new passage is created between anterior chamber (A/C) and subconjunctival space (Fig. 8.11) or sometimes between A/C and subscleral space (Fig. 8.12) so that the obstruction to aqueous outflow at angle of A/C is bypassed. There are many types of filtering operations such as trabeculectomy, Scheie's, cyclodialysis, sclerectomy, iridencleisis and trephining.

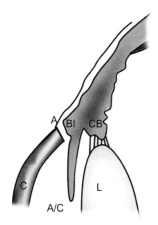

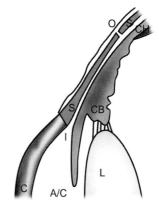

Figure 8.11: Basis for filtering surgeries such as trabeculectomy, Scheie's and trephining. New Channel (A) is created between anterior chamber (A/C) and subconjunctival space. BI – Site of block to aqueous drainage. CB – Ciliary body. C – Cornea. L – Lens

Figure 8.12: Another basis for filtering surgery such as cyclodialysis. New communication (I to O) is made between A/C and suprachoroid (subscleral) space. S – Sclera. CH – Chorid. CB – Ciliary body. C – Cornea. L – Lens

Trabeculectomy

It is indicated when medical treatment has failed to control raised intraocular pressure in glaucoma cases.

After application of speculum and superior rectus suture, conjunctiva is cut 6 mm from limbus and a limbal based conjunctival flap is reflected down. (Fornix based flap also is employed). The sclera is dissected off the Tenon's capsule. A square (4 × 4 mm) or a triangular partial thickness, limbal based scleral flap is reflected upto and beyond the limbal blue line. A 3 mm long and 2 mm broad limbal tissue containing deeper sclera and trabecular meshwork is removed. Peripheral iridectomy is done. Superficial scleral flap and conjunctival flap sutured. Scleral flap suture, if needed, can be releasable (Figs 8.13i to vi).

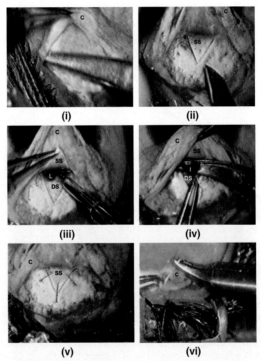

Figure 8.13: Steps of trabeculectomy operation. (i) Cutting of conjunctiva (C). (ii) Triangular shaped superficial scleral flap (SS) marked. (iii) The limbal tissue (L) punched out. (DS – Deep scleral area). (iv) Portion of peripheral iris (I) is cut after lifting up superficial scleral flap (SS). (v) Superficial scleral flap sutured. (vi) Conjunctival wound closed

Scheie's Operation

This surgery was once popular. It is indicated in medically uncontrolled glaucomas. Under a limbal based 4 mm conjunctival flap, the limbal tissue is incised for a length of 3 mm to 1/3rd depth. The posterior lip of wound is cauterised. The cut deepened still more minimally and posterior lip again cauterised. This is repeated till A/C is entered. Peripheral iridectomy done and conjunctival wound closed with running suture. Limbal wound is NOT sutured.

Cyclodialysis

It is indicated in aphakic glaucoma and in failed filtration procedures. Conjunctiva is cut for 5 mm about 10 mm from limbus at superotemporal quadrant. A 3 mm cut is made in sclera 7 mm away and parallel to limbus. Cyclodialysis spatula inserted via this incision into suprachoroidal (subscleral) space till the tip of spatula appears in anterior chamber. The spatula is rotated up and down so that ciliary body is detached for about 180° and a communication is established between anterior chamber and suprachoroidal (subscleral) space. Conjunctival wound closed.

3. Sac Surgeries

1. *Dacryocystectomy (DCT).* It is done for chronic dacryocystitis a) in older individuals, b) with ipsilateral impending intraocular surgery or c) ipsilateral corneal ulcer, and d) when sac is focus of infection such as of trachoma or tuberculosis, e) and in tumors of sac (Fig. 8.14).

   Anaesthesia is by infiltration of the sac region. Skin over sac is incised for about 1" starting 2 mm above the medial palpebral ligament and 3 mm medial to inner canthus. Orbicularis oculi and periostium over sac incised. The exposed sac is dissected free and removed. The nasolacrymal duct curetted. Wound is closed in two layers.

2. *Dacryocystorhinostomy (DCR).* It is done for chronic dacryocystitis especially in younger patients and in congenital dacryocystitis when other methods have failed. (It should be avoided for children below 3 years of age) (Fig. 8.15).

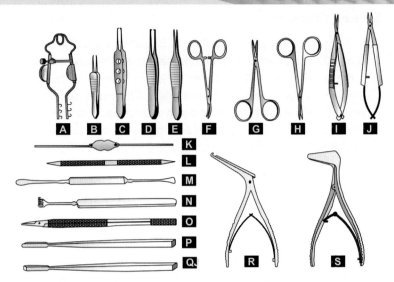

Figure 8.14: Instruments for DCR and DCT. A – Mueller's Lacrimal Sac retractor. B – St. Martin suturing forceps. C – Jaffe tying forceps (Straight). D – Fixation forceps (1 X 2 teeth). E – Wills hospital utility forceps. F – Halsted mosquito forceps (Curved). G – Eye scissors (Curved). H – Stevens tenotomy scissors (Curved). I – Westcott tenotomy scissors. J – Barraquer needle holder (Micro). K – Lacrimal probe set. L – Lacrimal dilator (Double end). M – Freer periosteal elevator. N – Knapp lacrimal sac retractor. O – Castroviejo blade breaker. P – Bone gouge. Q – Bone chisel. R – Kerrison bone punch. S – Nasal speculum

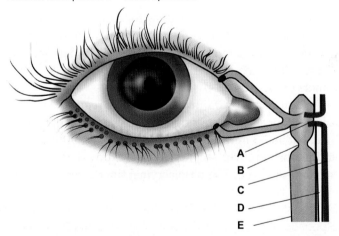

Figure 8.15: Principle of DCR. Opening (A) from sac into nasal cavity is created by punching out the in between bone (D) and suturing the newly created flaps of sac (B) and nasal mucosa (C) together

The anaesthesia is same as above. In addition, the nasal mucosa is anaesthetised with spray and ipsilateral nasal cavity packed with gauze. The incision is same as for DCT. After exposing and isolating the lacrymal sac, the lacrymal bone (of lacrymal fossa) is punched out. The nasal mucosa is seen. The exposed nasal mucosa and medial wall of sac are opened to form "I" shaped flaps. The flaps (or only the anterior flaps) of sac and nasal mucosa are sutured together through the opening in the lacrymal fossa. The skin wound closed in layers. Nasal pack is removed the next day. Syringing with antibiotic is done the next day and after one week. If DCR fails, conjunctivorhinostomy may be performed. In canalicular block, canaliculodacryocystorhinostomy is done.

In DCT, epiphora is not relieved. In DCR epiphora is cured. In acute dacryocystitis, surgery of any type (except incision and drainage of abscess) is NOT undertaken.

4. Enucleation

Although it can be done under regional anaesthesia, yet it is better to perform this surgery (and evisceration) under general anaesthesia (Fig. 8.16). After inserting the eye speculum, conjunctiva is cut all around out side the limbus. The Tenon's capsule is cut 3 mm behind limbus. The six extra ocular muscles are detached. The eye ball lifted up with enucleation spoon and the optic nerve cut with scissors as far behind as possible. The separated globe removed. Hemostasis obtained. Conjunctival and Tenon's wounds closed with or without an implant in the empty orbit. (Plastic implant such as Allen's can be buried in the orbit and Tenon's and conjunctiva closed over it separately).

5. Evisceration

After speculum insertion, the cornea is cut all around just *inside* (Fig. 8.17) the limbus and the intra ocular contents scooped out. It is important that all uveal tissue is completely removed. Hemostasis obtained. Tenon's capsule and conjunctiva wounds are closed separately. (Some surgeons do not close these wounds).

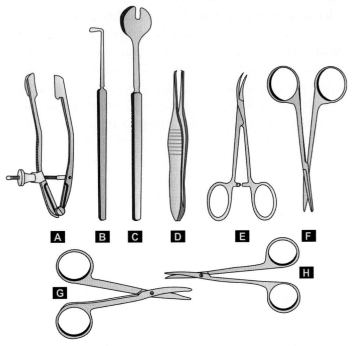

Figure 8.16: Enucleation instruments. A – Lancaster Eye speculum. B – Graefe muscle hook. C – Enucleation spoon.D – Elschnig fixation forceps. E – Halsted mosquito forceps (Curved). F – Eye scissors (Straight). G – Enucleation scissors (Curved). H – Tenotomy scissors (Curved)

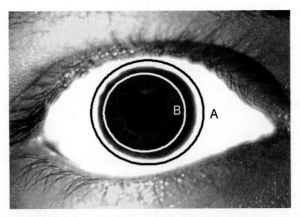

Figure 8.17: Incision sites for enucleation (A; just outside limbus) and for evisceration (B; inside the limbus in the cornea)

LASERS

Apart from incisional surgeries mentioned above, LASERS are used for treating certain ocular conditions. They are used for photocoagulation of retinal lesions, for iridotomy/capsulotomy, to lyse sutures, for trabeculoplasty and gonioplasty (Fig. 8.18).

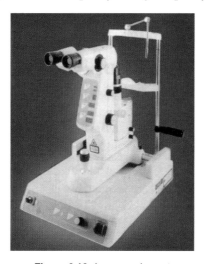

Figure 8.18: Laser equipment

SUTURES AND SUTURING

The word "suture" describes any strand of material used to ligate (tie) blood vessels or approximate (bring close together) tissues. As ophthalmic nurse, she must be familiar with the various types of sutures and the needle types.

OPTIMAL SUTURE QUALITIES ARE

1. High, uniform tensile strength, permitting use of finer sizes.
2. High tensile strength retention *in vivo*, holding the wound securely throughout the critical healing period, followed by rapid absorption.

3. Consistent uniform diameter.
4. Sterile.
5. Pliable for ease of handling and knot security.
6. Freedom from irritating substances or impurities for optimum tissue acceptance.
7. Predictable performance.

MONOFILAMENT AND MULTIFILAMENT STRANDS

Sutures are *CLASSIFIED* according to the number of strands in them. Monofilament sutures are made of a single strand of material. They encounter less resistance as they pass through tissue than multifilament suture material. They also resist harboring organisms. Crushing or crimping of this suture type can create a weak spot.

Multifilament sutures consist of several filaments twisted or braided together. This gives greater strength, pliability and flexibility. It may also be coated to help them pass relatively smoothly through tissue and enhance handling characteristics.

Sutures can be *grouped into* ABSORBABLE and NON-ABSORBABLE SUTURES.

I. *Absorbable sutures* are those that undergo rapid degradation in tissues, losing their tensile strength within 60 days. Absorbable sutures may be used to hold wound edges in approximation temporarily, until the wound has healed sufficiently to withstand normal stress.

Although they offer many advantages, absorbable sutures also have certain inherent limitations: 1) If a patient has fever, infection, or protein deficiency, it may accelerate suture absorption causing too rapid a decline in tensile strength, 2) if the sutures become wet or moist during handling, prior to being implanted in tissue, the absorption process may begin prematurely, 3) patients with impaired healing are often not ideal candidates for this type of suture.

II. *Non absorbable sutures* generally maintain their tensile strength for longer than 60 days. These are those which are not digested by body enzymes or hydrolysed in body tissue. They are walled off by body's fibroblasts. They are grouped into three classes: Class I – Silk; monofilament or braided. Class II – Cotton or linen. Class III – Metal–monofilament or multifilament.

ABSORBABLE SUTURES	
Suture	*Details*
Surgical Gut Plain, Chromic, Fast Absorbing	Submucosa of sheep intestine or serosa of beef intestine. Of collagen; monofilament. Absorption: Plain–70 days; chromic–90 days. Tensile strength: Plain–10 days; Chromic–21 days.
Polyglactin 910 Uncoated (VICRYL) and Coated	Copolymer of glycolide and lactide coated with Polyglactin 370 and calcium stearate. Braided suture. Absorption : 8 weeks.Tensile strength in 3 weeks - 40%
Polyglactin Acid	Homopolymer of glycolide
Poliglecaprone 25 (MONOCRYL suture)	Copolymer of glycolide and epsilon. Monofilament. Tensile strength: 2 weeks.Not used in eye surgery.
NON-ABSORBABLE SUTURES	
Suture	*Details*
Surgical Silk	Raw silk from silkworm. Twisted or braided. Should be used dry. Tensile strength lasts for one year.
Stainless Steel Wire	Specially formulated iron-chromium-nickel-molybdenum alloy. Monofilament or multifilament.
Nylon (Ethilon)	Polyamide polymer. Degrades by 20% per year. Monofilament knot needs more throws.
Polyester Fiber Uncoated (MERSILENE) Coated (ETHIBOND)	Polymer of polyethylene terephthalate. Coating is by polytilate. Remains in tissue indefinitely.
Polypropylene (PROLENE)	Polymer of propylene. Biologically inert. Used in infected area.

The numbers assigned to sutures depend on the size (diameter) of the suture. This differs if the number has a '0' attached to it. For example, number 4 size suture is thicker than number 2 size. At the same time 4/0 suture is thinner (smaller) than 2/0 suture. In eye surgery suture thicker than 4/0 is usually not used and the thinnest used is 11/0 (Fig. 8.19).

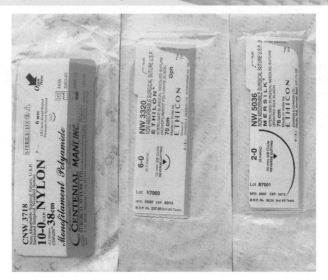

Figure 8.19: Certain frequently used suture materials. 10 – 0 is finer than 2 – 0

Ligatures

A suture tied around a vessel to occlude the lumen is called a ligature or tie. It may be used to effect hemostasis or to prevent leakage. Correct method in knot tying is important.

Ophthalmic Surgery

The eye tissues vary in blood supply and healing properties. Full thickness corneal wounds heal slowly. In cataract incisions, sutures should remain in place for approximately 21 days. Suturing of muscle to sclera requires sutures for about seven days.

Nylon was the preferred suture material for ophthalmic surgery. While nylon is not absorbed, progressive hydrolysis of nylon *in vivo* may result in gradual loss of tensile strength over time. Finer absorbable sutures are currently used for many ocular procedures. If sutures are absorbed too slowly granuloma can occur. Too rapid absorption may be a problem in cataract surgery.

While some ophthalmic surgeons promote the use of a "no – stitch" surgical technique, 10/0 coated VICRYL (polygalactin 910) violet monofilament sutures offer distinct advantages. They provide the security of suturing immediately following surgery and eliminate problems of suture removal and related endophthalmitis. Polyglactin 910 sutures have proven more useful than surgical gut as they produce less cellular reaction.

The ophthalmologist has many fine suture materials to choose from such as vicryl, ethilon and prolene (monofilament).

SURGICAL NEEDLES

They are made of high quality stainless steel and as slim as possible without loosing strength. It should be a) rust resistant, b) stable in the grasp of a needle holder, c) sharp enough to cut through, d) rigid enough to resist bending and e) be able to carry suture material through tissue with minimal trauma.

Various Types of Needles

Straight Needles

This shape may be preferred when suturing easily accessible tissue. They are not much used in eye surgeries.

Curved Needles

a. *Half Curved Needle*—The half curved or "ski" needle may be used for skin closure.
b. *Curved Needle*—Curved needles are used in eye surgeries. They allow predictable needle turnout from tissue. This needle shape requires less space for maneuvering than a straight needle. Needle holder is needed. The curvatures are 1/4, 3/8, 1/2, or 5/8 circle. These curvatures are measured in degrees –1/4 means 90° of a circle, 5/8 equals 225° and half circle equals 180° (Fig. 8.20).
c. *Compound Curved Needle*—The compound curved needle was originally developed for anterior segment ophthalmic surgery. It allows the surgeon to take precise, uniform bites of tissue. The 80° curvature of the tip becomes a 45° curvature throughout the remainder of the body. The initial curve allows reproducible, short, deep bites into the tissue. The curvature of the remaining portion of the body forces the needle out of the tissue, everts the wound edges and permits a view into the wound. This ensures equidistance of the suture material on both sides of the incision.

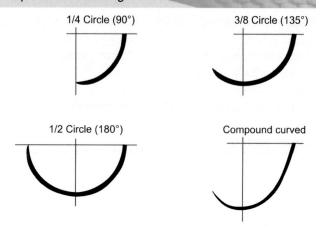

Figure 8.20: Shapes of some curved needles. The curvature notation is in relation to a circle and its degree (full circle is 360 degree)

Cutting Needles

Cutting needles have at least two opposing cutting edges. They are sharpened to cut through tough, difficult to penetrate tissue (Fig. 8.21).

a. *Conventional cutting needles*—It has a triangular cutting edge with the two cutting edges, on the side and a third cutting edge on the inside concave curvature of the needle. The shape changes from a triangular cutting blade to that of a flattened body.

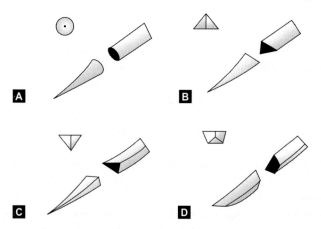

Figure 8.21: Shapes of certain needle points. A – Taper point. B – Cutting. C – Reverse cutting. D – Spatula type

b. *Reverse Cutting Needles*—They are used in ophthalmic surgery where minimal trauma, early regeneration of tissue and little scar formation are primary concerns. It has two side cutting edges and the third cutting edge is located on the outer convex curvature of the needle. This offers several advantages: i) More strength than similar sized conventional cutting needles, ii) tissue cutout is greatly reduced and iii) there is a wide wall of tissue on both the sides of needle track.

c. *Side cutting needles (Spatula Needles)*—They are flat on both the top and bottom, eliminating the undesirable tissue cutout of other cutting needles. The point is rhomboid shaped. They are designed for ophthalmic procedures. The needle separates or splits through the thin layers of sclera or corneal tissue.

Taper Point Needles

They are also known as round needles. It has a cone shaped point. They spread tissue without cutting it. The needle body then flattens to an oval or rectangular shape.

Blunt Point Needles

Blunt point (BP) needles dissect friable tissue rather than cutting it. They have a taper body with a rounded, blunt point that will not cut through tissue.

KNOT-TYING

The *type of knots* used can be
1. *Square knot:* Most frequently used method. Usually both the hands are used to tie. If incorrectly applied, it is liable to slip out.
2. *Surgeon's (friction) knot:* The first throw is twice, over which a single throw is made. The first throw does not slip even without holding it down. So this type of knot is mostly used in eye surgeries.
3. *Deep tie:* Used in tying something deep in body cavity.

The *method of tying* a knot is classified into:
1. *Instrument tie:* It is one in which tying is done with instruments and not with fingers. This is mostly employed by eye surgeons.
2. *Double hand tie.*
3. *Single hand tie.*

CHAPTER

9

Sterilisation

The word sterilisation brings to one's mind the asepsis of the operation theatre and its related materials.

Certain *TERMS* need explanation at this stage:

Antisepsis—Acting against and inhibiting growth of microorganisms (not necessarily killing them).

Asepsis—Absence of microorganism and freedom from infection.

Aseptic technique—Method of avoiding contact with microorganism.

Contamination—Infection by microorganism.

Disinfectant—An agent that kills growing or vegetative forms of bacteria. Those which act against M. tuberculosis (this has a waxy envelope), virus and fungus must specifically labeled.

Disinfection—Destruction of most of micro organism. It can be high level, intermediate level and low level disinfection.

Sterile—Free of microorganism and spores.

Terminal sterilisation—Procedure of destroying microorganism in OT or in other areas of patient contact at the end of the operation.

MONITORING THE STERILISATION

There are many ways to monitor that the sterilisation is properly carried out:
1. *Mechanical indicators*—A steriliser has many gadgets, recorders, thermometer and other devises. Maintenance and following the manufacturer's instructions are must.
2. *Biologic indicators*—The indicator is spore of bacteria inside ampule or strips. The exposed one to the sterilisation process and a control are checked after the sterilisation process. If the exposed one has no microbe growth but the control has, then the indicator is reliable.
3. *Chemical indicators*—The indicator tape or label may be outside the package or inside. If the desired reaction is not seen in the indicator, then the material is unsterile and cannot be used.

4. *Administrative monitoring*—Perfect supervision and correct procedures can assure proper sterilisation.

CLASSIFICATION

Sterilisation methods are classified into:

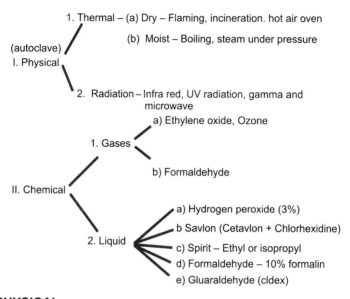

1. Thermal – (a) Dry – Flaming, incineration. hot air oven
   (b) Moist – Boiling, steam under pressure

(autoclave)
I. Physical

2. Radiation – Infra red, UV radiation, gamma and microwave

II. Chemical

1. Gases
   a) Ethylene oxide, Ozone
   b) Formaldehyde

2. Liquid
   a) Hydrogen peroxide (3%)
   b Savlon (Cetavlon + Chlorhexidine)
   c) Spirit – Ethyl or isopropyl
   d) Formaldehyde – 10% formalin
   e) Gluaraldehyde (cldex)

PHYSICAL

Thermal

Dry Heat Sterilisation

Dry heat is useful in sterilising equipments with cutting edge, metal containers and glass ware. It is able to go through items that cannot be penetrated by steam. Longer time is required and the duration of sterilisation itself differs. If done for much longer time, it may damage materials.

The *ovens* can be

a. *Mechanical convection oven.* It is usually an electrical one which has a blower. The usual cycle is 190°C for 12 minutes.

b. *Gravity convection oven.* The oven has two vessels. Steam is let in the outer chamber. The air in the inner chamber is heated and by gravity settles to the bottom. The temperature reached is around 120°C.

Moist

Boiling

This method may be effective for certain bacteria. But it may not be useful against bacteria with spores. Spores can resist boiling at 100°C for many hours. Boiling may be ineffective against certain virus. So this is not the ideal method for obtaining total sterility.

Pasteurisation with chlorine agents at 80°C for 30 minutes kills bacteria without spores.

Steam Sterilisation

Autoclave: It is useful in sterilising metal instruments, glass ware and culture media (Figs 9.1 and 9.2).

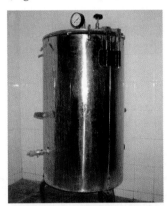

Figure 9.1: Vertical autoclave

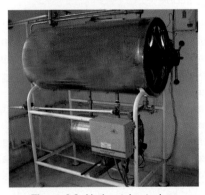

Figure 9.2: Horizontal autoclave

Here steam enters the autoclave chamber at high pressure wetting the materials. Moisture and heat combination is good at sterilising the items. The pressure itself has no effect on the microbes. The items need to be properly packed, free of grease and steam must come into contact with all the areas of the items. The steam itself must be pure. Autoclave may be vertical or horizontal.

In *gravity displacement sterilisation*, the steriliser has two shells. The steam enters in between the two and displaces the air already in it (as well as inside the inner shell) downwards. This air goes out of the steriliser. The steam fills up the chamber and the temperature goes up. The usual cycle is 120°C at a pressure of 18 pounds per square inch.

In *prevacuum steriliser*, air is almost removed from the inside of the steriliser and then the steam is let in. The steam is able to get to the interior of the materials to be sterilised. The articles are exposed to 132°C at 22 pound square inch for 4 to 10 minutes depending on the material.

In between surgery, quick sterilisation can be done with *flash* (134°C for 5 minutes) *or high speed autoclave* (120°C at 15 pounds per square inch for 15 minutes).

Steam sterilisation is not possible for materials that are steam sensitive. The organic materials must be thoroughly cleaned, materials washed and dried well. Drapes must be loosely packed. Impervious materials such as gloves or rubber sheets should not be folded. Flat packages are placed vertically, rubber goods are placed on edge and basins are placed on their sides. The sterilisation timing starts when the desired temperature is reached.

Radiation

Ultraviolet Radiation

This method is used for sterilising gloves, suture,bandages, cotton, plastic wares, facia lata and parenteral solutions.

The radiation (wave length 240 to 480) causes damage to nucleic acid and proteins of the organisms. It is effective against certain vegetative bacteria, virus and fungus. Its usefulness is limited. It is useful for eliminating air borne microorganisms in the OT. This radiation can cause skin damage.

Microwave is used to sterilize one or only a few instruments. It is faster (30 seconds).

Gamma rays from Cobolt-60 are usually employed in industries. In medicine it is used to sterilise disposable items such as gloves, syringe and catheters.

CHEMICAL

Gases

Ethylene Oxide (EO)

The materials that can be sterilised by radiation can be sterilised by EO. Sharp instruments can also be sterilised by this agent.

It is effective against microbes and their spores. It must have direct contact with the material. It is useful to sterilise items that are heat or moist sensitive. Exposure time is from 30 minutes to 2 hours at a humidity of 40 to 80 % and at a temperature of 60°C. The effect of EO depends the concentration of EO.

This gas is highly flammable. It irritates the mucous membrane and long-term contact can cause cancer. It does not penetrate metal or glass. It takes longer time to sterilise and requires expensive equipments. The materials must be dry (including the lumen of tubes). Aeration (exposure to air) should be done after sterilisation is over.

Ozone Sterilisation

It is used for plastics and metals. It takes about 5 hours to sterilise and takes place in four stages. It is an alternative for EO sterilisation. It is inexpensive and can be used for heat sensitive materials. It cannot be used for natural rubber material. It is harmful if inhaled.

Liquid

It should be remembered that most of the *liquid* sterilising agents do not kill the spores. This important point must be kept in the mind.

Hydrogen Peroxide

Metallic and non-metallic items which do not come into direct contact with the operative field are sterilised by this agent.

It is effective against bacteria, fungus and virus. It uses the plasma technology. Since this is effective at low temperature, heat sensitive items are sterilised by this agent. Only low temperature is required.

Alcohol

Sterilisation of suture and the skin of patient can be done with this agent. It will dissolve the cement used in lensed instruments.

Isopropyl alcohol (75 to 90 %) is effective against certain bacteria, viruses like hepatitis and a few fungi. It is not effective against hydrophilic viruses. The contact time should be 10 to 15 minutes. Longer contact causes hardening of plastic tubing. It can be used for wiping wire cords and to sterilise certain equipments. It is ineffective on evaporation.

Formaldehyde

It is useful in sterilising the theatre atmosphere. This agent irritates the skin and eyes. It should be thoroughly washed away before the instrument is used. It should not be used for rubber materials.

It damages protein of microbes. It is used as 37% in water (formalin) or as 8% formaldehyde in 70% isopropyl alcohol. It is an effective disinfectant and kills bacteria and fungus after 5 minutes contact, and virucidal after 10 minutes contact. It can destroy spores after 12 hours contact.

Glutaraldehyde (Cidex)

Plastic, rubber items, sharp instruments and lensed instruments (should not be used for long time) can be sterilised.

It is used as Cidex activated alkaline 2.4% dialdehyde, as Cidex (O.55%) orthophthalaldehyde (OPA) or as cidex (5.75%) OPA. They are effective against virus, bacteria and fungus after 10 minutes exposure (at 20°C). It is sporicidal after 10 hours exposure. It remains active in the presence of organic matter. Items must be dried before cidex is used. Fumes may be irritant.

Cetrimide is not used nowadays as it is ineffective against Gram-negative organisms.

Phenolic compounds and chlorine compounds are used mainly as house hold disinfectant. The former may be used for a few instruments that do not come in contact with skin or mucous membrane.

DANGERS DUE TO STERILISING AGENTS

Ethylene dioxide (gas)—It is a cancer causing agent. It should not come in contact with skin.

Formaldehyde—It is toxic to respiratory tract. It is an allergy-producing and cancer-causing agent. It can affect liver.

Glutaraldehyde—It is not much toxic. The fumes may irritate the eye and nose.

Ultraviolet irradiation—It can cause skin burns and conjunctivitis.

PACKAGING

The packaging material should be economical, free of lint, toxic ingredient and should not have any tear or hole in it.

The material can be:

1. Woven fabrics which are also called as linen or muslin. It is of cotton. It must be hydrated before sterilisation.
2. Non-woven fabrics are of cellulose and rayon. Their special use is they form barrier against microorganisms.
3. Peel pouches. They have paper on one side and clear plastic film on the other side.

Instead of packing straight in the packaging material, the instruments can be placed in open trays which have perforated bottom and then wrapped. Rigid closed containers are also used for sterilising.

The packing may be done with two wrappers which is called as sequential wrapping or with single wrapper.

The package must a) have identification marks, b) not get damaged during sterilisation, c) protect the instruments against microorganisms after sterilisation, d) cover the items totally, and e) permit sterilisation process to act effectively.

METHOD OF STERILISING VARIOUS MATERIALS

1. *Cloth and blunt instruments*—Autoclaving for 30 minutes at 120°C at a pressure of 15 lbs per square inch is effective. In between surgery, quick sterilisation can be done with flash (134°C to 5

minutes) or high speed autoclave (120°C at 15 pounds per square inch for 15 minutes).

2. *Sharp instruments and glass materials*—Hot air is employed to sterilise these items. Gases like ethylene oxide or solutions like glutaraldehyde (cidex), dettol or savlon is also used. Instruments are kept in these agents for 30 minutes. Cidex destroys spores. The chemical agent must be washed out before using the instrument. Cetrimide is not used nowadays as it is ineffective against gram-negative organisms. Spirit does not kill viruses.

3. *Laser lenses*—They are sterilised by ethylene oxide for one hour at a temperature of 55°C. They should not be steam autoclaved or boiled.

4. *Trays, furnitures, electrical cords*—They are wiped with alcohol.

5. *Rubber and plastic items*—A 2% aqueous solution of Glutaraldehyde is effective. Gas sterilisation and radiation are also effective.

6. *OT atmosphere*—Ultraviolet radiation and formalin fumigation.

7. *Skin*—Soap, chlorhexidine, iodine (including povidone-Iodine) and alcohol. Soap is effective mainly against Gram-positive organisms. While rinsing, the bacteria are removed mechanically.

10

Instruments

Identification, preparation and sterilisation of common ophthalmic instruments are very important for a nurse to be of good assistant in the operation field.

1. *PREPARATION OF INSTRUMENTS* for surgery is important. Once an operation is over, the instruments are collected in a designated place.

   a. The instruments are first *cleaned*. This starts with the scrub nurse who cleans the instrument as soon as the instrument's use is over. She wipes off blood and keeps them open. Once the instruments leave the sterile field, the circulating nurse gets them in a basin.

   b. She *immerses* them for a short period preferably in a proteolytic enzymatic detergent.

   c. The instruments are then *washed* with water.

   d. The instruments are *cleaned* with fine brush. For ophthalmic instruments this mechanical cleaning is preferred over automated washer-decontaminator/steriliser.

   e. *Ultrasound* cleaning is done for instruments with serrations and hidden holes. After this the instruments are cleaned in warm water. This method does NOT sterilise the instruments.

   f. The instruments are finally *washed* with distilled water.

   g. Instruments with moving parts are kept in bath containing water soluble *lubricants* for one minute. They are then drip dried. In some centers lubricants are applied before storing. But this lubricant has to be wiped off before sterilizing the instruments again.

   h. The instruments are then *inspected* for their fitness to be used again for operations.

   i. The instruments are *packed* for sterilisation. The heavy instruments must be packed separately from finer ones. The cutting edge of the sharp instruments must be protected against damage.

2. *DISINFECTION* is carried out. This is done both after use and immediately before use. The disinfectant is grouped into chemical and physical agents. The chemical disinfectants belong to alcohol, aldehyde, phenol and halogens. Physical disinfectants include boiling and ultraviolet radiation.

Points to be observed while using chemical disinfectant are:

a. The agent must be effective against bacteria and virus.

b. The period of immersion in the agent must be strictly followed.

c. The disinfectant agent must be washed off after the immersion period is over. The level of sterility after washing depends upon the sterility of the water used for washing.

(Details of the sterilisation techniques, disinfectants and methods available to sterilise the various materials are given under "Sterilisation" chapter).

Certain instruments of common uses are mentioned here (Figs 10.1 – 10.8). Specialised equipment such as phaco, vitrectomy and lasers are not covered.

Nurses must keep in her mind that there are so many *modifications or types* of one particular instrument and a surgeon is liable to use one particular instrument which may differ from that of another surgeon. A nurse must keep this in her mind.

Nowadays ophthalmic instruments have a dull surface. A polished, bright surface of the instrument may reflect the light and produce glaring especially under microscope. Microsurgery instruments are usually about 5 cms in length.

Nurse herself must be able to perform minor procedures such as suture cutting under microscope.

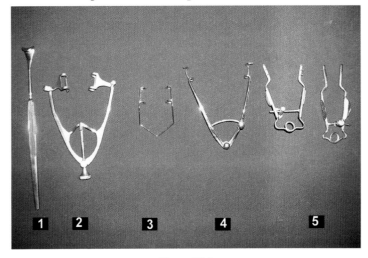

Figure 10.1

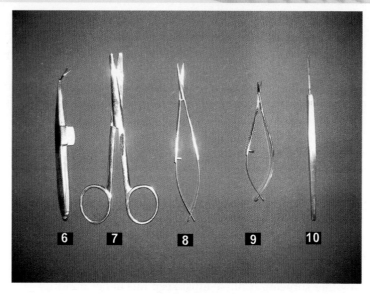

Figure 10.2

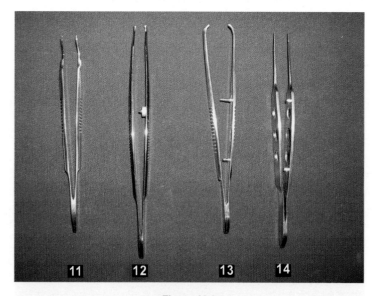

Figure 10.3

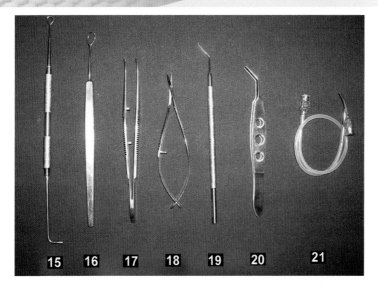

Figure 10.4

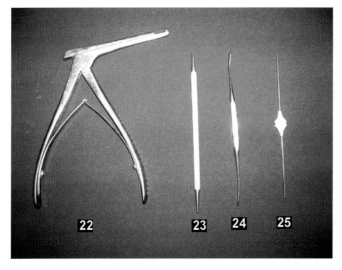

Figure 10.5

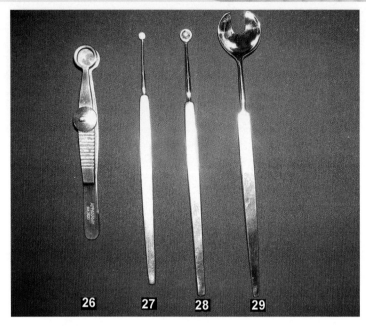

Figure 10.6

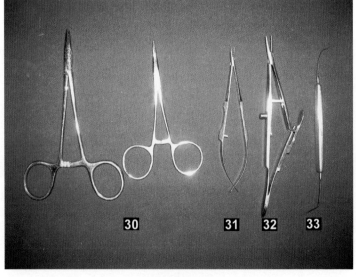

Figure 10.7

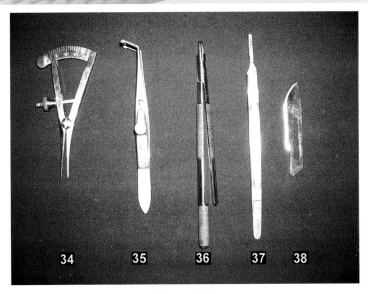

Figure 10.8

Figures 10.1 to 10.8: Certain instruments of common uses

1. *Desmarre's Lid retractor:* It has curved blades at the tips. It is useful in opening eyelids carefully a) while examining children, in non co-operative adults, for patients with severe blepharospasm, when there is danger of corneal perforation or in cases with severe edema of lids. b) For double eversion of upper lid. c) It may be used while removing exterior sutures of eye globe or any foreign body of cornea and conjunctiva. It is used to retract different tissues during extra ocular surgeries.

2. *Park Eye speculum:* The arms of the speculum are separated by the screw system. The opened lids cannot be closed so easily by the patient. It is used for separating the eyelids during all extra ocular operations like foreign body removal, excising pterygium, squint surgeries, evisceration and enucleation (removal) of eyeball.

3. *Wire speculum:* It is used for separating the eyelids during all extra ocular operations like foreign body removal, excising pterygium, squint surgeries, evisceration and enucleation of eyeball. It is preferred because of its lightweight. Some surgeons use this even for intra ocular surgeries.

4. *Lang Universal eye speculum:* This is also used for the above purposes. It is heavier and cannot be used in surgeries where eye ball is opened. It is called universal because same instrument can be used for both eyes.

5. *Muller's self retaining hemostatic lacrymal retractor:* To retract the lips of the skin wound in operations on sac like DCT and DCR. It has hooked, teeth like structures at its front arm. It acts as hemostat as well as retractor of wound lips.

6. *De Wecker's iris scissors:* It has a dove tail like cutting portion in the front. Spring action keeps the blades apart. It is used a) to cut (and excise) the iris as in foreign body in iris, cyst in iris, in traumatic prolapse of iris which is infected, various types of iridectomy like peripheral (button hole), sector, broad basal & optical (key hole) iridectomy, b) to cut iris at the pupil and c) in certain antiglaucoma operations. (Indications for each type of iridectomy–see under "iris forceps").

7. *Enucleation scissors:* It is a curved, long, comparatively heavy scissors used for cutting optic nerve during enucleation (removal of eye). It has blunt tips.

8. *Conjunctival scissors:* It is a delicate scissors with sharp tips. It is used for a) cutting the conjunctiva for limbal (or fornix) based conjunctival flap for cataract extraction (ab externo) or glaucoma surgery, b) pterygium excision, c) suture removal, d) squint surgery, e) detachment surgery and f) Gunderson's flap.

9. *Vannas corneal scissors:* It is a delicate scissors. It has sharp tips and is angled forwards.They are used for iridotomy, iridectomy, capsulectomy and to cut sclera in trabeculectomy.

10. *Von Graefe's cataract knife:* It is one of the sharpest instruments in the whole surgical field. It has a narrow blade with cutting edge on one side. The tip is sharp and pointed. It is used a) in cataract surgery section. Other uses are: b) Paracentesis, (opening the anterior chamber for evacuation of large, fluid, persistent pus or blood, in threatening corneal ulcer perforation), c) Chalazion incision, abscess incision, d) in certain antiglaucoma operations, f) to make a scleral opening at pars plana for lensectomy.

11. *Iris forceps (HESS):* It has a double bend at the front end. The tip has teeth. The iris is held with this instrument while cutting the former during iridectomy.

    Types of Iridectomy and their indications:- a) Peripheral iridectomy–Along with corneal grafting, cataract and glaucoma surgeries and in first three stages of narrow angle glaucoma. b) Complete (sector) iridectomy–Along with cataract surgery, for extensive posterior synechiae (in iridocyclitis), c) Broad basal iridectomy d) Optical (key hole) iridectomy–Central leucoma and central, stationary, congenital cataract, e) Iris excision–Impacted foreign body in iris (especially chemically active one), infected iris prolapse and tumors of iris (amount of iris excised depends upon the size of the pathology).

12. *Dastoor's superior rectus forceps:* This instrument resembles iris forceps; but is a heavier one. It also has teeth at its tips which are z-shaped. It is used to hold superior rectus tendon while applying suture under the tendon. This superior rectus suture gives control over the globe in surgeries such as cataract extraction, anti-glaucoma and keratoplasty. It enables surgeon to rotate the eye ball down. Eye ball is rolled down since most of the eye surgeries are done in the upper quadrant of globe.

13. *Fixation forceps (Graffe):* This instrument is a heavy, straight one and has teeth at its tips. Useful in fixing the globe and steadying it at limbus at 6 O'clock position while making incision at the limbus in cataract surgery, while performing paracentesis, antiglaucoma operations and discision. Globe is held at limbus since it is the site where conjunctiva and sclera are adherent. So a firm grip can be obtained.

14. *Corneal forceps:* Forceps are grouped into toothed tissue forceps which are used to grasp the tissues and non-toothed tying forceps used for tying sutures. Corneal forceps is a toothed one for holding the corneal/limbal tissue, especially while applying suture.

15. *Lens hook or lens expresser (with vectis):* This is a two-in-one instrument. On one side (the curved end) is lens hook and at the other end (having a circle) is the vectis. The lens hook is

used to a) apply pressure and rupture the zonules of lens in the lower part in the intra capsular cataract surgery, b) express the nucleus (and cortex) out in extra capsular cataract extraction, and c) hold extra ocular muscles during enucleation (removal) of eyeball. d) It may be used in squint operations.

16. *Lens Loop (Levies):* To remove subluxated or dislocated lens. (This instrument is also known as **vectis**). Irrigation type is used in extra capsular cataract surgery.

17. *Arruga's Intracapsular forceps:* It has a cup at the inside of both its tips. Useful in holding the anterior capsule of lens and delivering the lens in toto in intracapsular cataract extraction (ICCE). The lens capsule is held at 12 O' clock or at 6 O' clock position. It is also used to remove capsular remnant after unexpected rupture of lens capsule in ICCE. Lens (in intra capsular cataract extraction) can also be removed completely using cryo equipment, vectis or erysiphake.

18. *Gills-Vannas Capsulotomy scissors:* It is a delicate scissor. It is used to cut pieces of lens capsule tags. It has sharp tips.

19. *Sinskey lens hook (dialer):* At its tip it has a small bend with blunt tip. It is used for rotating the Intraocular lens (IOL) after the latter is placed inside the capsular bag. The IOL is rotated so that the haptics (the arms) are placed horizontally.

20. *Faulkner Lens holding forceps:* This instrument is used to hold the IOL (by the haptics or optic) while introducing it into eye. The arms do not have any teeth. Another type of lens holding forceps is the one like a blade holder.

21. *Simcoe cannula:* It has irrigation - aspiration ports at one end and the other end has the facility to attach to a syringe. The aspiration canula opening size is from 21 G (0.5 mm) to 23 G (0.3 mm). It is employed to separate epinucleus from nucleus of lens and to aspirate out the cortical matter in extracapsular cataract extraction. It can be reverse type also.

22. *Bone punch (Kerrison):* The tip has cutting edge which slides over a base. The tip sizes are from 0 (1 mm) to 3 (4 mm) sizes. Used to punch out an opening in the lacrymal bone in dacryocystorhinostomy operation. Through this opening

made in the bone the sac and nasal mucosa are joined together to create a bye pass (new) channel for the tear to flow directly from sac to nasal cavity.

23. *Nettleship's punctum (lacrymal) dilator:* To dilate the punctum a) before syringing and probing the nasolacrymal passage and b) in congenital atresia of punctum. c) It may be used as a marker for retinal detachment and squint surgeries. The tip sizes are 1 (small) to 3 (big).

24. *Lacrymal dissector with curette (Lang):* Dissector side of the instrument is used to dissect and isolate sac during dacryocystectomy (DCT) and dacryocystorhinostomy (DCR). Curette end of the instrument is used to curette the nasolacrymal duct in DCT. It can be used to open nasolacrymal duct. The epithelial remnant is scooped out after DCT with this instrument.

25. *Lacrymal probe (Bowman):* The probe has blunt end. The sizes range from 0000 to 4. a) To probe the lacrymal canaliculi in congenital dacryocystits b) To investigate the site of obstruction in chronic dacryocystitis. c) To identify sac during DCR and DCT.

26. *Chalazion clamp (or forceps):* One arm has a flat plate and the other arm has a round or oval opening. The diameter of the opening is from 8 mm to 12 mm (round model) to 20 mm (oval model). Useful in fixing the chalazion mass during surgery. Flat plate of the instrument should be on the skin side and the opening on the conjunctival aspect.

    Vertical incision is made in the conjunctiva. This is to prevent cutting other neighboring ducts as well as blood vessels–both run in vertical direction.

    The usefulness of this instrument in the operation: a) It forms a base for operation, b) prevents bleeding, c) helps in everting the lid, d) protects the eye and e) steadies the lesion. (In an older person, if chalazion recurs at the same site after surgery, one has to consider carcinoma).

27 and 28. *Chalazion curettes:* These instruments are used to curette out the contents of chalazion after the swelling is opened by a vertical incision on the conjunctival aspect.

29. *Enucleation spoon (Wells):* It has kidney shaped cup like tip with cleavage at the end. It is used during enucleation (removal) of the eyeball.

    Indications for enucleation: Retinoblastoma (cancer of retina) and malignant melanoma (in stages I and II), in sympathetic ophthalmia, blunt trauma with total dissolution of eye, painful blind eye such as absolute glaucoma, bleeding anterior staphyloma, for eye bank purposes, phthisis bulbi (shrunken blind eye), long standing total retinal detachment with severe photopsia. This surgery is not done in panophthalmits.

    Usefulness of this instrument during the surgery: a) To pull up eyeball (so as to perform long stem enucleation), b) to protect eyeball while cutting optic nerve with scissors and c) to steady eyeball while cutting optic nerve.

30. *Artery forceps (Straight and Curved):* This is also known as hemostat. It usually has a box lock, jaws, shank and ratchets. The ratchets help in locking the instrument after catching the tissue/blood vessel. It may have straight or curved jaws. It is used for some extraocular surgery and in sac surgeries.

31. *Needle holder (without lock):* Eye surgeons never hold needles with fingers. They always grasp them with needle holder. Needle holders are either locking or non locking; straight or curved. Needle holder without lock is used more often than one with lock.

32. *Needle holder (with lock):* This is comfortable when the surgeon wants to concentrate more on the operation area and does not want to be disturbed by holding onto the needle himself. But the surgeon must remember that he is using a needle holder with lock.

33. *Iris Repositor (Dastoor):* It has narrow flat blades at both ends which are malleable (can be bent). Used to replace the prolapsed iris back into anterior chamber a) during eye operations and b) in early traumatic iris prolapse if it involves the lower quadrant and is free of dense infiltration. c) For paracentesis (draining the anterior chamber).

34. *Caliper:* To measure distances. It is used in squint and retinal detachment operations.
35. *Jameson muscle forceps:* The jaws have 4 to 6 teeth. It has slide lock. It is useful for holding the extraocular muscle during squint surgery. The slide lock locks the two jaws together so that the detached muscle during squint and retinal detachment surgeries caught by this instrument does not slide out.
36. *Blade breaker:* This is used to break blades into small pieces. It is also used to hold the blade piece while cutting.
37. *Bard Parker blade handle:* These are reusable handles made of brass. Handle sizes are 3, 4 and 7.
38. *Bard Parker blade:* These are disposable blades made of carbon steel. There are two types – Ten series : Blade sizes are known as 10, 11, 12 and 15. They fit handle size numbers 3 or 7. Twenty series : Blade sizes are 20, 21, 22, 23, 24 and 25. They fit handle size 4. The blade shown here is size 22.

CARE OF INSTRUMENTS

The instruments that are used in ophthalmology are broadly grouped into those that are used during surgery (blunt and sharp instruments) and those office equipment that are used as ancillary ones and have lenses including lasers. (Operating microscope comes under this category)

I. SURGICAL INSTRUMENTS

At the end of operation (after the count is over) the non disposable instruments are washed first with running water. (The nurse should wear gloves during such washing). Each instrument is then cleaned separately. Using a baby toothbrush is ideal for instruments which have hinges (such as needle holder, scissors). Such hinged instruments should be opened wide and the hinges cleaned of all blood and tissues. They are then dried and packed. The tips and cutting edge of the sharp instruments must be protected. They are sent for sterilisation.

II. OFFICE EQUIPMENT

Certain *basic rules* must be followed while dealing with these instruments:

1. The lenses and mirror in the instrument should be wiped clean with lint-free cloth or it should be left to the specially trained technicians.
2. The bulbs should not be touched with bare fingers. Tissue paper must be used. To remove dust or finger prints from the bulbs, lint free clothe must be used.
3. When not in use, the equipment must be stored/kept in the case or well covered (larger equipment).
4. Before dealing with complicated equipment, the operations manual must be gone through thoroughly.
5. An instrument which has lenses in it should be lubricated only by specialist.

Dust over the *LENSES* are removed with the help of air blown on it with bulb syringe, lens brush or with lens cleaning paper. Ordinary tissue paper, paper lint and kerchiefs should not be used. It can be further cleaned using a cotton ball wet with lens cleaning fluid or clear dish washing fluid. Remove the cleaning fluid and dry the lens with lint-free absorbent lens cloth. A dry lens should not be rubbed. Dismantling the lens assembly should never be attempted. The surfaces of the lens that are seen only are to be cleaned. Thorough cleaning of lens should be done periodically by the experts.

For those lenses that come in contact with patient's eye, they can be sterilised by using 2% glutaraldehyde or ethylene dioxide. The disinfectant should be wiped clean with lint-free absorbent lens cloth. Lenses should not be autoclaved (except a few made specially for OT purpose) or boiled.

The applanation tonometer is cleaned with alcohol and allowed to air dry for 5 minutes. The prism head can also be removed and soaked in 3% hydrogen peroxide for 5 minutes, rinsed under running water and allowed to dry by itself.

Maintenance of *LASERS* should be attended to only by experts. The nurse should not handle lasers without studying the manual. She should never handle them carelessly.

Ocular
Therapeutics

Pharmacology is science of study of drugs. Nurse should know the basic of certain important drugs used in ophthalmology.

I. MYDRIATICS

These drugs dilate the pupil. *Phenylephrine* (2.5%) is the most commonly used one. Mydriatics are of special use to dilate the pupil in the study of fundus and in improving vision in certain cataract cases. Some of the mydriatics such as *atropine* and *homatropine* paralyse the ciliary muscle also (*cycloplegia*). With cyclopegics there is some amount of defective distant vision and gross reduction in near vision (reading, etc). Cycloplegic-mydriatics are used for treating corneal ulcer, iridocyclitis, to check vision in children and in certain postoperative conditions.

These drugs may be grouped into short acting (tropicamide and cyclopentolate) and long acting (atropine and homatropine) compounds.

Side effects of these drugs include stinging, glaring and defective vision. When applying atropine (and homatropine), the lacrymal sac area should be pressed for one minute so that the drug does not go into nasolacrymal duct, get absorbed via nasal mucosa and produce systemic problems. These drugs should never be used in a narrow angle glaucoma case.

II. MIOTICS

They cause constriction of pupil and contraction of the ciliary muscle. These result in improvement of vision (in visual field) and reduction in ocular pressure. Miotics are used to constrict pupil during refraction after it is dilated, in glaucoma cases and in certain accommodative squints. Examples of miotics are pilocarpine, physostigmine and carbachol.

III. CHEMOTHERAPY

Chemotherapy is the use of drugs to kill or to inhibit the growth of infectious organisms or cancerous cells. (This topic deals only with chemotherapy for infectious agents).

Antibacterial agents

They can be bactericidal (kills the bacteria) or bacterostatic (prevents growth of bacteria). They are obtained from soil microbes or by chemical synthesis.

1. Sulfa

It was discovered in 1935 as a by-product of dye industry. The various sulfas that are in use are Mafenide, silver sulfadiazine (both for burns cases), Sulfacetamide (for eye infection), Sulfamethizole and Sulfamethoxazole (for urinary tract infections).

Sulfa drugs are mainly bacterostatic only. In trimethoprim–sulfamethoxazole combination, the former is bactericidal and the latter is bacterostatic.

They are *effective* against all cocci (except *streptococcus*), certain bacilli (*B. coli, C. diphtheriae, Claustradium*), fungus (nocardia, actinomyces), virus (PLT) and toxoplasma gondii. Sulfones and diamox are certain derivatives.

Adverse reactions: Agranulocytosis (vitamin B_6 is administered), hematuria, anuria, nausea, vomiting, cyanosis, Stevens-Johnson syndrome, polyarteritis nodosa and drug fever. Prolonged use can result in macrocytic anaemia.

2. Antibiotics

They can be classified as follows:

A. BETA LACTAM GROUP

    a. Penicillin – Penicillinase sensitive and resistant
    b. Cephalosporins

a. Penicillin: Penicillin was discovered by Alexander Fleming (1929) and first used clinically by Henry Florey (1948). It is obtained from penicillium mould. It can be grouped into:

1. *First generation*—They mainly act against Gram-positive organisms and Neisseriae. These can be—
    i. *Penicillinase sensitive:* They are destroyed by acid, alkalis, metals and rubber. They are Penicillin G and penicillin V.
    ii. *Penicillinase resistant*: They are cloxacillin, methicillin and oxacillin.

2. *Second generation*—They are Penicillinase sensitive. Examples are amoxicillin and ampicillin. They are effective against Gram-negative and Gram-positive organisms.
3. *Third generation*—They are also penicillinase sensitive and are effective against *Pseudomonas* and *Proteus* group of bacteria. Carbenicillin is one drug of this group.
4. *Fourth Generation*—They are effective against *Pseudomonas*, *Proteus* and *Klebsiella*. These drugs are penicillinase sensitive. Sodium ingestion is less. Piperacillin belongs to this group.

Clavulanic acid inhibits penicillinase. It has been combined with amoxycillin.

Adverse Effects

These include allergy (serious), nausea, rashes and diarrhoea. In very high doses it can produce convulsions.

Ampicillin in chronic lymphatic leukemia can cause rashes due to interaction with abnormal lymphocytes.

Third generation penicillin can produce sodium or potassium excess (sodium in the drug) and is dangerous in cardiac patients.

Chloramphenical and tetracycline are incompatible with penicillin.

b. Cephalosporins: Discovered in 1945 from sewage of Sardinia Island. It has B-lactase ring (like penicillin).

They interfere with bacterial cell wall synthesis. They are used mostly for Gram-negative bacteria. They are bactericidal. They are mainly useful for patients with penicillin allergy and for infection with certain Gram-negative organisms. Cephalosporinase breaks down cephalosporin molecule.

They are given either orally (cephalaxin, cephadroxil, cephradine, cephaclor) or parenterally.

The Side Effects

These include hyper sensitivity (lesser than penicillin), nephrotoxicity (more with aminoglycosides) and false positive Benedict's and Coomb's test. Intravenous injections can produce local inflammation or phlebitis. Oral route can cause gastrointestinal upset.

B. AMINOGLYCOSIDES

Streptomycin, the first aminoglycoside, was isolated from chicken throat and from heavily manured field by Wakeman in 1943. Drugs of this group include amikacin, gentamicin, streptomycin, kanamycin and neomycin.

They are poorly absorbed from gastrointestinal tract (so only given by intravenous or intramuscular routes) and excreted almost unchanged in urine.

They are used mainly against Gram-negative bacilli. They are bactericidal.

Adverse reactions: Orally, they cause nausea, vomiting and diarrhoea. By injection, they cause nephrotoxicity and (temporary) ototoxicity. Albuminuria and oliguria may occur. Deafness may become permanent if used for longer period. Other reactions are malar paraesthesia, contact dermatitis (with streptomycin) and drug fever.

It causes neuromuscular block. So general anaesthesia can cause respiratory arrest during surgery due to diaphragmatic paralysis. Combination with cephalosporin increases nephrotoxicity.

C. TETRACYCLINES

They were first isolated by Duggar and Subba Rao (1947). First one to be isolated was chlortetracycline. The others are oxytetracycline, doxycycline, tetracycline and methacycline.

They are bacteriostatic by preventing protein synthesis. But also involve the host causing anabolic effect. They are useful against Gram-positive and Gram-negative infections. They are of special use in rickettsiae and *Vibrio cholera* organisms.

Adverse Reactions

1. Thrush, moniliasis and sore throat due to suppression of normal flora. (B complex given).
2. Dental enamel hypoplasia and pigmentation of teeth (forming calcium orthophosphate). These drugs are not advised for children.
3. Effect on bone growth is very minimal.
4. Rarely, intracranial hypertension and liver and pancreatic damage.
5. Photosensitivity occurs with dimethylchlorotetracycline.
6. Fanconi syndrome (Polyuria, proteinuria and acidosis) when outdated products are used.

D. MACROLIDES

Erythromycin was the first one to be introduced. Roxithromycin, azithromycin, clindamycin, norfloxacin, ofloxacin and enoxacin are others.

They are available as estolate, succinate, stearate and glucoheptanate. They are destroyed by gastric acidity. Hence they are enteric coated.

These drugs are very useful against *staphylococcus, pneumococus, corynebacterium* and *treponema*.

Adverse reactions

They are very minimal and include nausea, vomiting and diarrhea. The may cause hepatitis.

E. POLYPEPTIDES

This group includes polymyxin, bacitracin, trycothricin. They are effective only against Gram-negatives.

Adverse reactions

They can cause gastrointestinal tract upset, ototoxicity and neurotoxicity.

F. LINCOSAMIDE

The drugs are clindomycin and lincomycin. They are *effective* against Gram-positive and anaerobic Gram-negative organisms.

Adverse reactions

Stomatitis, glossitis, anorexia, metallic taste, angio edema, vertigo, tinnitus, aplastic anaemia (with rapid Intravenous administration), cardiac arrest and hypotension, colitis and jaundice.

G. QUINOLONES AND FLUROQUINOLONES

They are bactericidal agents. They are effective against *staphylococcus, entero, pseudomonas, haemophilus* and *neisseria organisms*. They are less active against strepto and inactive against anaerobic bacteria.

The drugs of this group are: Nalidixic acid, ciprofloxacin, perfloxacin and ofloxacin.

3. Nitrofurantoin

Used in urinary tract infection. Oral dose is 100 mg qid.

Adverse reactions are gastrointestinal tract upset, neuritis, anaemia and allergic reaction (which can result even in pulmonary edema).

Fortified Drops

Sometimes, especially in corneal ulcers, the amount of antibiotic concentration in the drops should be more. For this, fortified drops are prepared. These drops are to be applied once in 2 minutes for 30 minutes and then ½ hourly. The concentrations are:

Gentamicin	14 mg/ml (80 mg to 5 ml commercial drug)
Tobramicin	10 mg/ml
Cephalosporidine	32 mg/ml (2 ml saline to 500 mg +13 ml tear substitute)
Penicillin G	33000 U/ml
Vancomicin	31 mg/ml

Antifungal Agents

It can be polyene antibiotics (such as nystatin, pimaricin) or non antibiotics compounds such as imidazoles and triazoles. Most of them act on the fungal cell wall rupturing it.

Antivirals

They suppress the viral multiplication. They are purine or pyrimidine derivatives. Adenine arabinoside (3% ointment), acyclovir and ganciclovir are purine derivatives. Idoxyuridine (0.1%) drops and Triflourothymidine (1% drops) are pyrimidine compounds. Zidovidine is used against HIV virus. They are of special use, as local agents, in herpes simplex and herpes zoster cases. Some of them like acyclovir can be given by systemic route also.

IV. CORTICOSTEROIDS

They are useful in inflammatory conditions. If the inflammation is due to infection, the latter should be controlled before corticosteroids are used. Commonly used steroids are cortisone (1%), hydrocortisone (1.5%), betamethasone (0.5%), prednisolone (1%) and fluoro-methalone (1%). Corticosteroids (cortisones) are combined with antibiotics in certain preparations used locally in eye. Indiscriminate use of local cortisone can result in cataract, rise in ocular pressure (glaucoma), overgrowth of bacteria, fungus or virus, delayed healing and lowering of resistance to infection.

V. NSAIDs

These are also anti-inflammatory agents which do not belong to cortisone family. These are safer than cortisones. They include diclofenac, flurbiprofen and ketoralac. They can be used for a long time without many side effects.

VI. ANAESTHETICS

(See under "Ocular surgeries")

VII. ANTIMETABOLITES

They are used to reduce the local fibroblastic activity (formation of fibrous tissue). The two important drugs are:
1. *Mitomycin C*—Daily use of it is advised as 0.4 mg/ml after pterygium excision to prevent recurrence. In antiglaucoma operation 0.4 mg/ml is placed for two minutes at the operation site.
2. *5 Fluorouracil*—In glaucoma surgery 50 mg/ml is placed under the conjunctiva during operation.

These two drugs are dangerous ones and must be handled and used with care and caution.

VIII. ANTIGLAUCOMA DRUGS

(See under "Glaucoma")

IX. OTHERS

Mast call stabilisers such as cromogen and olopatadine are effective against symptoms of itching and redness. They prevent release of histamine. They are of special use in vernal conjunctivitis.

Decongestants reduce redness of eye and give relief from irritation. They constrict the conjunctival vessels. Naphazoline is the most common decongestant used.

Lubricants are useful in symptoms of dryness of eye. Preservative free drugs are preferred. They basically contain methyl cellulose.

Dyes are used to stain certain ocular structures. Locally used ones are fluorescein (2%), rose bengal and congo red. They are used to study the fundus, lacrymal passage and to assess the intraocular pressure by applanation method (fluorescein), to study iris (Indocyanine green).

Enzymes—Hyaluronidase (used with local anaesthetic agents) is employed in ophthalmology. Alpha chymotrypsin and urokinase are not used nowadays.

Chelating agents that are used in ophthalmology are Ethylene diamine tetra acetate 0.7% (EDTA) (used to remove calcium from band shaped keratopathy of cornea) and Desferrioxamine mesylate 10% (to remove the rust stain of cornea after iron foreign body removal).

Antineoplastic agents such as fluorouracil (pyrimidine antagonist) and Mitomycin C (an antibiotic) are used in eye surgeries.

Certain other antineoplastic agents are used against retinoblastoma.

Adhesives are used to seal small irregular corneal tear, in certain lid surgeries, retinal detachment operation and epikeratoprosthesis. The agent used is cyanoacrylate.

ROUTES OF ADMINISTRATION

Medication for eye has to cross certain main barriers depending on the route of administration: Corneal epithelium (for locally applied drugs), blood-brain and blood-aqueous barriers.

I. *TOPICAL*—These are ointment, drops or inserts applied directly to the conjunctival sac. The drops do not stay in the eye for long and so require hourly applications. The ointments stay for longer time; but cause minimal blurring of vision. Inserts are like wafers. The drugs in it may be released even for as long as a week. Many of them which are soluble act for a few hours to one day only. Iontophoresis is not used often.

II. *LOCAL INFECTIONS*—The injection can be made under the conjunctiva, into anterior chamber (intracameral injection), into the vitreous or outside the globe (retrobulbar or periocular).

III. *SYSTEMIC ROUTE*—This route is employed if the disease is outside the eye in the orbit or lacrymal passage. It is also used to supplement the local therapy if needed. Entry into the eye by drugs by this method depends on the molecular size and its lipid solubility.

Intravenous and intramuscular are the other routes that are employed.

12

Microbiology

Microbes are grouped into bacteria, fungus, virus and parasites.

BACTERIA

Bacteria are single celled organisms which are essential to human life. Some of them reside inside the gastrointestinal tract and produce essential vitamin. Some others are found in tissues such as conjunctiva; but do not cause any harm normally. Some of them are useful to human beings. Many antibiotics are from bacteria.

Once there is a break in the protective layer of body, they enter the tissues and cause damage locally. They can get disseminated through blood to distant organs.

Most of bacteria which cause diseases are spherical shaped (called cocci), or rod shaped (called bacilli). Some have flagella and are motile. Some of them have endospores. These spores, in their resting phase, are difficult to kill by routine sterilisation methods. Once ideal conditions occur, the spores go back to active state. Spores are formed by Gram-positive bacilli only.

There are many ways of *grouping* bacteria. The simplest is by their staining character (colouring the microorganisms and cells by special stains and method). Method frequently used for bacteria is known as Gram's stain. Based on Gram's stain, bacteria can be grouped into Gram-positive (these bacteria are stained violet) or Gram-negative (stained pink).

Bacteria *cause disease* by the toxins they produce. These toxins include: a) Exotoxin (released by bacteria while they are alive). These are formed by Gram-positive bacteria. These toxins are very toxic. About 200 ml of botulism type A toxin can kill the entire world population. b) Endotoxin (released when the bacterial cell wall breaks and the bacteria die). They are produced mainly by Gram-negative bacteria. c) Heterogenous substances. These toxins can be of many varieties.

The *identification of bacteria* is by making a slide smear with the discharge and staining it with Gram's stain (or some other stain). Slide study is assisted by growing bacteria in culture media and studying the culture appearance. Most of the media contain agar. The media can either be solid or liquid.

Microorganisms are identified by:
a. Physical appearance
b. Its motility
c. Spores (if present)
d. Pigmentation (if present)
e. Staining (especially Gram stain)
f. Growth in media (solid or liquid)
g. Antibody testing
h. Biochemical activity

BODY'S DEFENCE MECHANISMS

1. *Phagocytosis*—Blood cells such as macrophages engulf the invading bacteria and kill them.
2. Anatomical protection such as skin, mucous membrane, closure of orifice.
3. *Immune system*—They are found in lymphatic system. They neutralise the toxins released by the bacteria. The important ones are autotoxin which act against exotoxin and antibodies which act on the endotoxin.
4. Antibody and inflammatory response.

Following are certain bacteria that cause diseases in human beings (Figs 12.1 to 12.5): Gram-positive cocci – Staphylococci, Streptococci, Pneumococci. Gram-negative cocci – Gonococci, Meningococci. Gram-positive bacilli – B. anthrax, *Clostridium*, *Corynebacterium diphtheriae*. Gram-negative bacilli – *Salmonella, Shigella, E. coli, Vibrio cholera*.

FUNGUS

They are either unicellular or multicellular aerobic organisms which grow in tissues.

They can be *grouped into* filamentous fungi, yeast (round in shape) and dimorphic. Many of them have thread like structure (hypha). Hypha may be septate (division is seen inside the hyphae) or non septate. Bunch of hypha which is like a mat from which

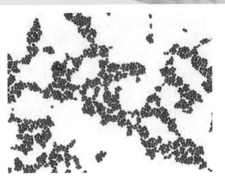

Figure 12.1: Staphylococcus. It is Gram-positive (Stained violet) and are in bunches like grapes

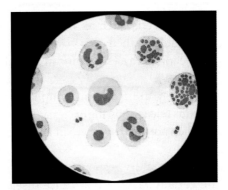

Figure 12.2: Gonococci. They are Gram-negative (stained red). They are in pairs

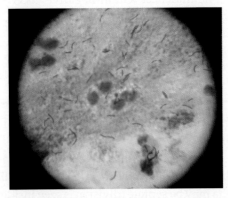

Figure 12.3: Mycobacterium. They are stained violet and are rod shaped (bacilli). They cause tuberculosis and leprosy

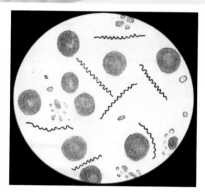

Figure 12.4: Treponema pallidum. (Organism causing syphilis). They are like cork screw

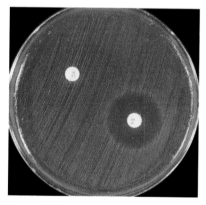

Figure 12.5: Antibiotic sensitivity test. Antibiotic discs are placed in the bacterial colony. Clearing around the disc means that the particular organism is sensitive to that antibiotic

hyphae project is known as mycelium. Fungi form spores which are usually at the tip of the hypha (Fig. 12.6).

Some important fungi are aspergillus, penicillium, candida, fusarium, cephlosporium, monilia and diplosporium.

Fungi are *identified by* the appearance of the spores and hyphal element in the slide preparation. The slide specimen is stained with lactophenol cotton blue or acridine orange. The fungus is grown in special media such as Sabouraud's medium or potato dextrose agar. It can be grown in test tube (Fig. 12.7) or in Petri dish (Fig. 12.8). The appearance of the culture is also helpful in identifying fungus.

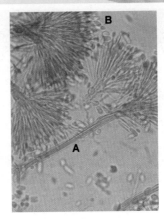

Figure 12.6: Fungal growth as seen in a slide culture. The spores (B) are present atop the hyphal element (A)

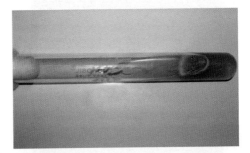

Figure 12.7: The appearance of fungal colony (green colour) in a test tube culture of Sabouraud's medium

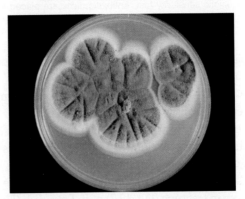

Figure 12.8: Fungal colony in a Petri dish medium. The colony is always studied from the front as well as from behind

They usually cause chronic infection. The inflammation is due to mycotoxin, proteolytic enzymes and soluble antigens.

VIRUS

They are submicroscopic organism which does not have its own metabolism. They are grouped into DNA virus and RNA virus. They are also classified on the basis of their replication mechanism.

The basic particle is called virion which has a nucleic acid core and a protein coat (capsid). Lipid envelope is seen in certain virus. From this lipid coat project spikes called peplomer (Fig. 12.9). The virus causing various diseases has many shapes.

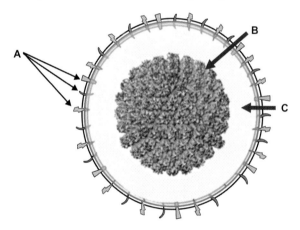

Figure 12.9: Virus. A – Peplomer. B – Nucleic acid core. C – Capsid

The viruses can be lipid viruses such as influenza, rubella, HIV and hepatitis B and are easily destroyed. Hydrophilic viruses are exemplified by polio virus and hepatitis A virus. These resist destruction by sterilisation more than lipid viruses. Knowledge of the group to which a virus belongs is important since a hydrophilic antiseptic agent may not be effective against lipid virus.

Important viruses are herpes simplex, herpes zoster, HIV, those of variola (small pox; now eradicated in the world), vaccinia, measles, mumps and varicella (chicken pox).

PROTOZOA

They are bigger than bacteria and many fungi. They are motile. They have their own reproductive cycle – either in living organism or in ordinary environment such as water. They are identified by their appearance. Malaria, toxoplasmosis, leishmaniasis, amebic dysentery and sleeping sickness are some of the diseases caused by protozoa.

HELMINTHS

This group of organisms are macroscopic ones. Some examples are hook worm, ascariasis, tape worm, filariasis and flukes. Each has got its own life cycle involving an intermediate and a definite host.

13

Spectacles and Contact Lens

SPECTACLES

HISTORY

Glasses of some sort were being used as early as 350 BC. History states that, in first century AD, Emperor Nero of Rome used glasses; but it might be tinted coolers for the weak eyes he had. Legend states that St. Jerome (5th century AD) invented glasses.

Abu – Ali al Hasan (of 10th century AD) was the first to study lenses, reflection, refraction and dispersion of light in detail. Reading stones of monks of Middle Ages were developed based on his study. The *glasses* as we know today were invented in 1250 AD. These were used mainly for reading purpose. Roger Bacon used the first 'real glasses' in 1268. Invention of printing popularised use of glasses. The glasses were so costly then that they were mentioned in wills by the dying ! Fitting of glasses was done by untrained vendors till the middle of 19th century. The range of choice was not wide. Glasses were available for aphakia, short sight and for "old sight" (Reading glass). Florence was leading in lens making. Glasses for reading were the first to be used. Benjamin Franklin invented the bifocals. By 19th century cylindrical lenses were introduced.

To begin with, lens *materials* were made of semiprecious stones (Fig. 13.1). Now it is never used. The material used is thinner if its refractive index is high. The common lens materials used now with their refractive indices are – plastic (1.4), high index plastic (1.60) high index glass (1.9), crown glass (1.35), flint glass (1.63) and polycarbonate (1.5).

Plastic lenses weigh less, do not break so easily as glass, need no hardening and can be tinted in various ways. But it is prone to be scratched easily and does not protect the eye from UV rays. The central thickness ranges from 2.0 to 3.0 mm. The glass lenses are hardened either by chemicals or by heat. Safety lenses are made from polycarbonate. Crown glasses are used for making photo chromatic lenses which darken when exposed to sunlight (UV rays). Polarised lenses are used in snow areas. Glass and plastic lens can be coated so that they are scratch resistant.

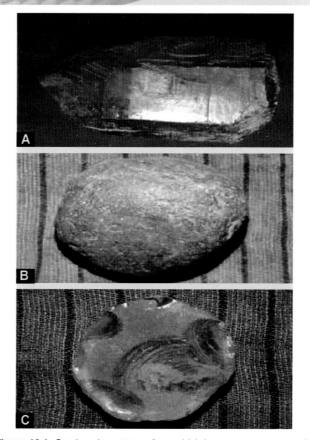

Figure 13.1: Semiprecious stones from which lenses were once made

The *trial case* was introduced in 1843. Jaeger introduced his test types for distance and near in 1843.

Spectacle frame was introduced in Italy by the end of 13th century; but it was not like the one we see now. It was present only around the lens and a handle was provided to hold it by hand. By 16th century bow spectacle which can be worn over the nose was introduced (Fig. 13.2). Germany was leading in making frames. To begin with lenses were mounted in leather, wood, horn, bone or light steel. The affluent used hand held spectacles with silver or gold frames. Hand held single lenses in decorative frames were popular and were used by Washington and Napoleon (18th

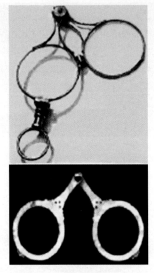

Figure 13.2: The type of frames that were used during the 19th century.

Century). Even then temple side arm was not known. The frames were secured to head gear even ! Ear rails were introduced by the beginning of 19th century.

The parts of spectacles frame are rim, nose pad, bridge and temple piece. The temple piece should not press on patient's temple area. Frame should be such that it should not keep sliding forward.

TYPES OF LENSES

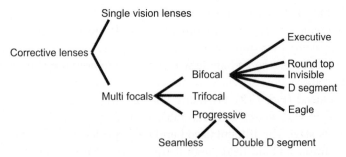

Single vision lenses are used usually for distance vision.

Bifocals are used for distance and near vision. The distance vision segment is at the top and the near vision segment is below. Rarely the near vision segment is above—This is dispensed for certain persons such as electricians who have to see small objects while looking up. The five types of bifocal are given below (Fig. 13.3).

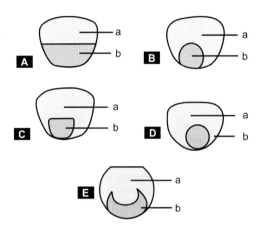

Figure 13.3: Types of spectacle lenses. Bifocals. A – Executive model. B – Round top type. C – D segment. D – Invisible (blended) bifocal. E – Eagle bifocal. a – For distance vision. b – For near vision

Trifocals help in focusing at far, medium and near distances. The top segment is for distance, the middle one for medium distance and the lower one is for near vision (below 33 cms). The types of lenses are the same as for bifocals (except eagle). It may be seamless type or double D type (Fig. 13.4).

In *progressive lens* the power starts from top (for distance vision) and changes slowly so that at the bottom is the area for near vision (Fig. 13.4).

The power of the lens in the spectacles is checked using *lensmeter*. It measures both spherical and cylindrical powers and the axis (direction of the prism power) of the latter (Fig. 13.5).

The nurse must see to it that the lensmeter is kept covered while not in use. The non optical portion of it should be kept clean by wiping it with cloth. Any dust over the lens surface must be blown off with a puff of air and then cleaned with soft lint free lens cloth.

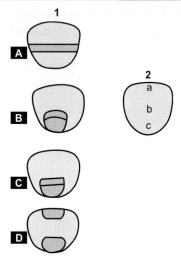

Figure 13.4: Trifocals. 1. A – Executive model. B – Round top type. C – D segment. D – Double D trifocal. 2 – Progressive seamless multifocal lens. a – For distance vision. b – For intermediate vision. c – For near vision

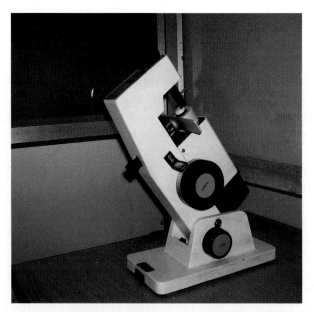

Figure 13.5: Lens meter. This is used to measure accurately the power of lenses in the spectacle

CARE OF SPECTACLE

A nurse posted in ophthalmology should know the following about spectacles as some patients might ask these points.

1. The lenses need cleaning with sprays and cloth. Simple soap and warm water are enough. Any soft cloth can be used to dry/clean the lenses. Plastic lenses tend to be scratched easily. So one should be careful with such lenses.
2. While not in use, the spectacles must be kept in such a way that the lenses are not touching any surface such as table or floor. The spectacles must be folded and temple piece must be down on the surface.
3. When not in use, it should be kept in the glasses case.
4. Some persons may find it difficult to adjust to bifocals in the beginning (the floor looks a bit nearer when seen through the near vision segment).
5. Many persons find adjusting to seamless progressive multifocal lens very difficult.

CONTACT LENS

HISTORY

It was Leonardo da Vinci who described first the idea of contact lens in 1508. In 1632, Rene Descartes suggested placing a lens on the eye. It was in 1887 that a German, FE Muller, produced the first glass contact lens. Soft contact lens was introduced in 1971 commercially. Rigid gas permeable lens was available by 1979 and extended wear soft lens in 1981. Disposable lenses were in the market by 1995 (Fig. 13.6).

CONTACT LENS MATERIALS

Hard contact lenses are made from PMMA; but these lenses are not popular now. They do not permit oxygen to pass through them to cornea. *Rigid gas permeable (RGP) lenses* permit oxygen to reach the cornea. These lenses are made from silicone, cellulose acetate butyrate and acrylate.

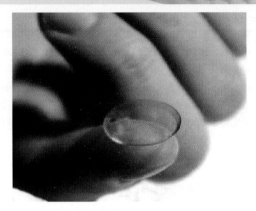

Figure 13.6: Contact lens

More than 4/5th of patients use *soft ("hydrophilic") contact lens* which is made from gel like hydrogel material. These lenses rarely cause spectacle blur. They are comfortable, easily adoptable, inexpensive and are available as disposable lenses. The disadvantages include less durability, expensive cleaning and more deposit formation.

RGP is preferred because it maintains corneal physiology, gives better vision because of larger optical area, has fewer spectacles blur and is easier to adopt with better comfort. But these lenses get scratched easily, fragile, have complicated cleaning procedure and are costly.

Extended wear lenses are either soft contact lenses or certain RGP lenses. They have high oxygen permeability. They can be worn for a week continuously.

Daily wear contact lenses can be worn for one day without removing.

Contact lenses are *worn for* cosmetic (fashion as well as restorative), toric purposes (for high astigmatism), as bifocals and for therapeutic uses (bandage lenses).

CARE OF CONTACT LENSES

A nurse must know the following facts:
1. Sterility is the most important one. The lens must be free of mucous, contaminant and microbes. Specific cleaning solution must be used.

2. Wetting agent is to be used. It acts as a buffer between the lens and cornea on one side and lens and lids on the other side.
3. They should be stored in the specific container – either dry or in storage solution.
4. While inserting and removing, the fingers must be clean.
5. Finger nail should not touch the lens.
6. Face make up should be done after putting on the lens
7. Right and left lenses should not be mixed up.
    1. Caution should be followed while using any eye drop when the lens is in the eye.
    2. Head spray, soap and cosmetics should not come into contact with contact lenses.

DISADVANTAGES

1. Redness, watering and discharge from the eye.
2. Irritation of eye. Lens needs cleaning or replacement.
3. Corneal edema, swelling, corneal vascularisation and even infection by *acanthamoeba* can occur.
4. Allergy is seen in about 1/6th of the patients. This is mostly caused by disinfectant fluid.
5. "Loss" of lens in the "eye".
6. Large papillae in the conjunctiva.

Table 13.1: Contact lens and spectacles		
	Contact lens	*Spectacle*
Correction of error	Better	Good
Correction in keratoconus	Possible	Not satisfactory
Image size	Almost normal	May be smaller or larger
Infection risk	Present	Nil
Maintenance	Required much	Almost nil
For sports persons	Ideal	Not very ideal
In dust and smoke	May not be ideal	No problem
Cost	More	Less

14

Community Ophthalmology

Community Ophthalmolgy is not so important for a nurse. At the same time she should be aware that the patient is part of the community, that he might having a problem which is part of the community and that this problem may have to be dealt with in the wider sense.

DEFINITION

Community ophthalmology deals with identification of common causes of ocular morbidity in different regions, assessing the needs of the population, selecting appropriate intervention strategies, planning education programmes and analysing the utilisation patterns.

MAGNITUDE OF VISUAL PROBLEM

According to World Health Organization (WHO) definition of blindness is visual acuity < 3/60 in the better eye with glasses correction. The number of people with visual impairment worldwide in 2002 was in excess of 161 million, of whom about 37 million were blind and 124 million people had low vision. It is estimated that 7 million people become blind every year and the number of blind people are increasing by 1-2 million per year. In India, a survey done in 2001-2002 revealed an overall prevalence of blindness to be 1.1% but in >50 years age group it rose to 8.5%.

CAUSES OF BLINDNESS

Cataract remains the leading cause of blindness in all regions of the world except for the most developed countries. It is responsible for 48% of world blindness, which represents about 18 million people. In India, cataract is contributing to 63.7% of blindness.

Glaucoma is the second leading cause of blindness globally as well as in most regions. Worldwide the number of persons estimated to be blind as a result of primary glaucoma is 4.5 million.

Corneal blindness is another major cause of visual deficiency. Trachoma is responsible for nearly 4.9 million blind. Every year some 40,000 go blind due to vitamin A deficiency. Now this has started coming down. Severe refractive errors have been estimated to account for about 5 million blind people worldwide. According to WHO, there are an estimated 124 million people in the world with low vision.

Prevention and Control Strategies

The *five levels* of prevention and intervention methods adopted are:
1. *Positive health promotion*: It is done through health education, environmental hygiene and healthy dietary nutritional practices.
2. *Specific prevention of diseases*: This can be achieved by providing Vitamin A supplementation to children and pregnant women as well as immunization against childhood diseases specially measles that has the tendency to precipitate Vitamin A deficiency. Adopting preventive methods for other diseases.
3. *Early diagnosis and treatment*: Conditions such as cataract and refractive error are more amenable to this approach where blindness can be identified at an early stage and cured through the help of spectacles and/or surgery.
4. *Disability limitation*: This is done by monitoring cases and treating them as in glaucoma and diabetic retinopathy where complete cure is not possible; but the extent of disability can be reduced to a considerable extent. It has to be combined with health education and awareness campaign for full utilisation of existing services.
5. *Rehabilitation:* It is needed for absolute and irreversibly blind cases that need social and economical support. This helps the blind people by building their capacity in various aspects of life so that they can lead a socially and economically productive life.

Programmes for Blindness Prevention and Control

I. VISION 2020: THE RIGHT TO SIGHT

It is a collaborative effort between the WHO, International Agency for Prevention of blindness (IAPB) and other non-governmental organizations (NGOs) and professional bodies. India has committed itself to the global initiative to reduce avoidable blindness. Target diseases are cataract, refractive errors, childhood blindness, corneal blindness, glaucoma and diabetic retinopathy.

II. NATIONAL PROGRAMME FOR CONTROL OF BLINDNESS (NPCB)

India launched the programme in 1976 as a 100% centrally sponsored one with the support of DANIDA. It incorporated in the earlier *Trachoma control programme* which was started in 1968. Its main objectives are to reduce the backlog of blindness, to develop eye care facilities in every district and to secure participation of Voluntary organisations in eye care. Eye camp approach was the main aim. Next step is establishment of permanent infrastructure – It is in *three tier system* – a) At *primary health center* by strengthening its equipments, b) At *district level* to deal with cataract, glaucoma, lid lesion and emergency care of eye injuries and c) At *central institution* to deal with retinal detachment, corneal grafting and glasses treatment (tertiary eye care). It is in medical colleges and in regional institutes of ophthalmology.

III. OTHER SPECIFIC PROGRAMMES

1. *Trachoma control:* GET 2020 (Global Elimination of Trachoma) was launched under WHO's leadership in 1997. Through this programme control activities are instituted through primary health centers. Trachoma control programme was launched in India in 1963. Later this was incorporated into NPCB.
2. *School eye health services:* Six to 7% of children aged between 10 and 14 years have problems with their eye sight affecting their learning at school. Health education is an important part of the school health services. Students should be taught to practice the principles of good posture, proper lighting, avoidance of glare etc.
3. *Vitamin A prophylaxis:* Children are most vulnerable to this form of malnourishment. Vitamin A supplementation, immunisation against measles, nutrition education and avoidance of harmful traditional practices are carried out. Under the Vitamin A distribution scheme in India 200, 000 IU of Vitamin A is given orally to all children between the ages of one to 6 years every 6 months.

4. *Occupational Eye Health services:* This programme helps to prevent/treat eye hazards in industries.

District Blindness Control Societies (DBCS)

The concept of District Blindness Control Societies was born due to a need to decentralise National Programme for Control of Blindness (NPCB) for the implementation of the programme.

The *3 tier system* is followed in DBCS. Primary Health Centers (PHC) form the first tier. District hospital and medical colleges form the second and third tiers.

Mobile units are the backbone of DBCS (and NPCB). They function at district level and at central level (of 3 tier system).

HEALTH EDUCATION

Health education is very important for a nurse. She may have to give this in outpatient wing or in ward. It a) Makes the patients and the relatives realize the importance of preventive aspects of blindness such as Vitamin A deficiency, use of irritants to eye and injury to eye. b) Imparts to the people the basic concepts of various eye problems such as the cataract, glaucoma, etc. c) It educates the people to utilize the various schemes of Government. d) It is able to clear many wrong concepts and superstitions about eye and its problems.

Health education can be given whenever an opportunity for it arises. Nobody is exempt. Even general physician and surgeons may not be aware of many a thing in ophthalmology.

BLIND REHABILITATION

The blind rehabilitation can be *grouped* into three headings:
1. *Orientation and mobility training*—With orientation and mobilisation training, a blind is able to move around freely in his own house, surrounding area and, if possible, to distant places. The use of cane and use of seeing-eye dog come under this category.

2. *Vocational training:* The blind is given vocational training so that he can earn his own livelihood, become a useful member of the community and regain his own confidence and dignity. Occupations taught are cane work, weaving and tailoring. But blind are employed by many companies nowadays and the work of ORBIT in this field is laudable. Managing of telephone booths is a useful occupation for the blind.

   Another vocational training is teaching of Braille letters.

3. *Normalisation:* It is the final stage of rehabilitation. Home training is instituted at this stage so that his family and society accept him as a useful, normal citizen.

15

Glossary

Abrasion: A scratch.

Abscess: A localized collection of pus surrounded by inflamed tissue.

Acute: Refers to a condition that flares up suddenly and persists for only a short time.

Adnexa : The tissues and structures surrounding the eye; includes the orbit, extraocular muscles eyelids, and lacrymal apparatus.

AIDS: A vial infection.

Anaesthetic: A drug that causes temporary deadening of a nerve.

Anterior segment: The front of the eye; includes the structures between the front surface of the cornea and the back of lens.

Antibiotic: A drug the combats a bacterial infection.

Aqueous humor: The clear fluid that fills the anterior chamber.

Arc perimeter: A device that can test the entire field of vision.

Aseptic technique: A range of procedures to prevent the spread of infectious microbes.

Bacteria (Singular: bacterium): Single celled microorganism; some bacteria are capable of causing disease in humans.

Blind spot: The sightless area in the normal visual field corresponding to the optic disc.

Canal of Schlemm: A structure that drains the aqueous humor from the anterior chamber.

Canthus: The point where the upper and lower eyelids meet.

Cautery: The application of an electric current or heat to destroy a lesion and prevent bleeding.

Chronic: Refers to a condition that has persisted for some time.

Complication: A problem that occurs during or after medical or surgical treatment/or disease.

Concave lens: A piece of glass or plastic in which one or both surfaces are curved inward. Also called negative lens or minus lens.

Cone: The retinal photoreceptor largely responsible for sharp central vision and for colour perception.

Confrontation field test: A test comparing boundaries of the patient's field of vision with that of the examiner.

Congenital: Refers to many disease processes or effect that is present from birth.

Contraindication: Any condition that renders a particular treatment, medication, or medical device inadvisable for a particular patient.

Convex lens: A piece of glass or plastic in which one or both surfaces are curved outward. Also called positive lens or plus lens.

Corneal topography: A photographic procedure that produces a colour coded "map" of the surface of the cornea.

Cycloplegia: Temporary paralysis of the ciliary muscle (preventing accommodation).

Cylindrical lens: A lens that has curvature in only one meridian.

Decongestant: A drug that constricts the superficial blood vessels in the conjunctiva and reduce eye redness.

Dendritic: Branch-shaped, such as the corneal ulcers seen after infection with the herpes simplex virus.

Descemet's membrane: The thin, elastic layer between the corneal stroma and the corneal endothelium.

Developmental: Refers to any disease process or effect that results from faulty development of a structure or system.

Diabetes mellitus: A condition in which the body is unable to produce enough insulin, the hormone required for sugar metabolism.

Diabetic retinopathy: A progression of pathologic changes in the retina caused by long standing diabetes mellitus.

Diagnosis: Determination of a medical condition.

Dilator muscle: The iris muscle that dilates the pupil.

Diopter: The unit of measure of the power of a lens.

Diplopia: Double vision.

Direct ophthalmoscope: A hand-held instrument with a light and mirror system that affords an upright, monocular view of fundus.

Disease: A specific process in which abnormal changes result in malfunction of a particular part or system of the body.

Diverge: To spread apart

Edema: Swelling caused by a large amount of fluid in a part of the body.

Emmetropia: The refractive state of an eye that is able to focus objects correctly on the retina.

Empiric treatment: Starting of medical treatment based on probable cause, before test results confirm a diagnosis.

Endocrine system: The body system consisting of multiple glands that produce chemicals called hormones.

Endophthalmitis: A serious ocular bacterial infection with inflammation of the vitreous and adjacent tissues.

Esophoria: The inward deviation of the eye that is present only when one eye is covered.

Esotropia: The inward deviation of the eye even when eyes are uncovered.

Etiology: The cause of a disease.

Exo deviation: The outward deviation of the eye.

Exophoria: An outward deviation of eye which is seen if one eye is covered.

Exotropia: The outward deviation of the eye even when eyes are uncovered.

Floaters: Small particles of dead cells, debris or degenerative matter that become suspended in vitreous. They appear as spots.

Fluorescein: A dye used for diagnosis of corneal and retinal conditions.

Fornix: The loose pocket of conjunctival tissue where the eyelid and globe portions of the conjunctiva meet.

Fovea: The center of the macula in the retina.

Fundus: A collective term for the retina, optic disc, and macula.

Fusion: The blending by the brain of the separate vision images received by the two eyes.

Genetic: Refers to a trait that is inherited from either or both parents.

Germicide: A chemical that kills germs

Globe: The eye, without its surrounding structurers. Also called eyeball.

Gonioscopy: A method of viewing the chamber angle through a special contact lens placed on the anesthetized eye.

Gram staining: The procedure for identifying by staining bacteria and certain other microbes according to their reaction to a dye.

Hemianopia: The type of visual field defect in which the right or left half of the field in one eye is missing.

Hemostasis: The control of bleeding.

Herpes simplex virus: A type of virus that infects the cornea, producing branch – like ulcers (dendritic keratitis).

Homonymous hemianopia: The type of visual field defect in which the right or left-half of the field in both eyes is missing.

Host: The animal or plant from which a microbe gains nutrients and the conditions necessary for its survival and reproduction.

Immune reaction: The body's response to infection, in which antibodies are manufactured to neutralize the microorganism.

Incision: A cut produced by a sharp instrument.

Indentation: A form of tonometry in which the amount of corneal indentation produced by a fixed weight is measured.

Indirect ophthalmoscope: An instrument that affords an inverted but wider view of the fundus than does the direct ophthalmoscope.

Infection: The invasion and multiplication of harmful micro-organisms (bacteria or fungal) in the body tissues.

Inflammation: A local protective tissue response to infection, in which specialized cells move to the affected area.

Informed consent: The process by which, after discussion with the doctor/surgeon about the risks and benefits of a proposed procedure, the patient agrees to undergo a treatment.

Insert: The delivery system by which a drug containing wafer is placed on the conjunctiva under the upper or lower eyelid

Iridotomy: A type of laser surgery to make an opening in the iris.

Ischemia: A condition in which the supply of blood to a part of the body is severely reduced.

Kinetic perimetry: Type of perimetry that uses a moving test object.

Leceration: A cut.

Legal blindness: A best-corrected visual acuity of 20/200 or less or a visual field reduced to 20" or less in the better-seeing eye.

Lesion: An abnormal tissue or a break in a normal tissue.

Limbus: The junction between the sclera and the cornea

Lubricant: A medication that helps maintain an adequate tear-film balance or keeps the external eye moist.

Malignant: Refers to any tumor that is cancerous and has the capacity of spreading to other parts of the body.

Metabolism: The physical and chemical processes by which the body converts food into energy and new body tissues.

Metastasis: The process by which cancerous cells move to other parts of the body and produce new tumors.

Microorganism: An extremely small life form invisible to the unaided eye. Also called microbe.

Miotic: A drug that causes the iris sphincter muscle to contract, producing miosis (pupillary constriction).

Mold: A form of fungus that produces a woolly, fluffy, or powdery growth.

Neoplasm: A new growth of different or abnormal tissue.

Neovascularisation: The abnormal growth of new blood vessels.

Nystagmus: A condition in which the eyes continually shift in a rhythmic side to side or up and down motion.

Ocular media: The three transparent optical structures that transmit light- cornea, lens and vitreous.

OD: Latin for right eye.

Optic radiation: The nerve fibers that transmit visual information from the lateral geniculate body to the visual cortex.

Optic tract: The part of the visual path way between the optic chiasma and the lateral geniculate body.

Orthophoric: Refers to the absence of visual deviation; normal.

OS: Latin for left eye.

Pachymeter: An instrument, attached to a slit lamp, that measures the distance between corneal epithelium and corneal endothelium.

Palpebral fissure: The almond shaped opening between the upper and lower eyelids.

Palsy: Paralysis

Perimetry: The measurement of the expanses and sensitivity of peripheral vision and the visual field.

Peripheral vision: The visual perception of objects that surround the direct line of sight.

Pharmacology: The study of the medicinal use and actions of drugs.

Phoria: The tendency of the eyes to deviate; usually prevented by the brain's effort to fuse the two images.

Photocoagulation: Surgical welding with laser light beams.

Photorefractive keratectomy (PRK): A type of refractive surgery that employs laser light to reshape the corneal curvature.

Placido disk: A flat disk with alternating black and white rings encircling a small central aperture, used in checking the regularity of the anterior curvature of the cornea.

Pledget: A small tuft of cotton soaked in an anesthetic solution for application to the conjunctiva and punctum.

Plus lens: See convex lens.

Polymethylmethacrylate lenses: Contact lenses that permit oxygen to reach cornea.

Posterior chamber: The space between the back of the iris and the front of the vitreous; lens is suspended in this chamber.

Posterior segment: The rear portion of the eye; includes the vitreous and the retina.

Presbyopia: The progressive loss of the accommodation due to aging.

Proptosis: A condition characterized by a protruding eyeball. Also called exophthalmos.

Pseudophakia: The use of an intraocular lens (IOL) to correct the vision of an aphakic patient.

Radial keratotomy (RK): A type of refractive surgery in which radial incisions are made in the cornea to flatten its curvature.

Refraction: The process of measuring a patient's refractive error and to determine the optical correction needed.

Refractive error: A pathologic deficiency in the eye's optical system.

Retinoscopy: The procedure to detemine a refractive error.

Rubeosis iridis: A condition in which the iris develops neovascularization.

Slit lamp (biomicroscope): An instrument used for close examination of the lids and lashes and anterior segment of eye.

Snellen chart: A printed visual acuity chart consisting of specially formed alphabets arranged in rows of decreasing letter size.

Spherical lens: A concave or convex lens whose curvature is uniform.

Spherocylinder: Also simple cylinder. A combination of a spherical lens and a cylindirical lens. Sometimes called toric lens.

Static perimetry: The type of perimetry that uses a stationary target that can be varied in size, brightness, and position.

Strabismus (Squint): A misalignment of the eyes that may cause vision to be disturbed.

Symptom: A subjective complaint by patient that indicates a disease.

Synapse: The connection between nerves, where electric impulses are transmitted.

Syndrome: A set of signs or symptoms that is characteristic of a specific condition or disease.

Tear film: The moist coating (composed of 3 layers) that covers the anterior surface of the globe.

Topical application: The delivery system by which a drug is applied directly to the surface of the eye or surrounding skin.

Transparent: Refers to a substance that permits the passage of light through it without obstruction.

Trauma: A wound or injury to the body from outside the body

Triage: The screening of patient (in person or by telephone) to classify them into three categories.

Trial frame: The frame into which various trial lenses are placed; used during refraction.

Trial (lens) set: A box containing a set of various lenses which are introduced before a patient's eye to select the corrective lens.

Tropia ("squint"): A condition in which misalignment of the eyes is present even when both the eyes are uncovered.

Varicella-zoster virus: A herpes virus that produces chicken pox and the skin disease zoster (shingles).

Vehicle: The inert liquid in which a drug is dissolved to form a solution.

Visual cortex: The area of the brain responsible for the conscious registration of vision; destination of nerve impulses from retina.

Visual field: The height and breadth of space seen by the eye when the vision is fixed straight ahead.

INDEX